FELICITY CLARK

VOGUE GUIDE TO SKIN CARE, HAIR CARE AND MAKE-UP

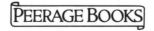

PEERAGE BOOKS

First published in Great Britain in 1981 in three separate
volumes by Penguin Books Ltd

This edition first published in 1982 by
Allen Lane

Published in 1987 by
Peerage Books
59 Grosvenor Street
London W1

ISBN 1 85052 097 6

Printed in Hong Kong

Contents

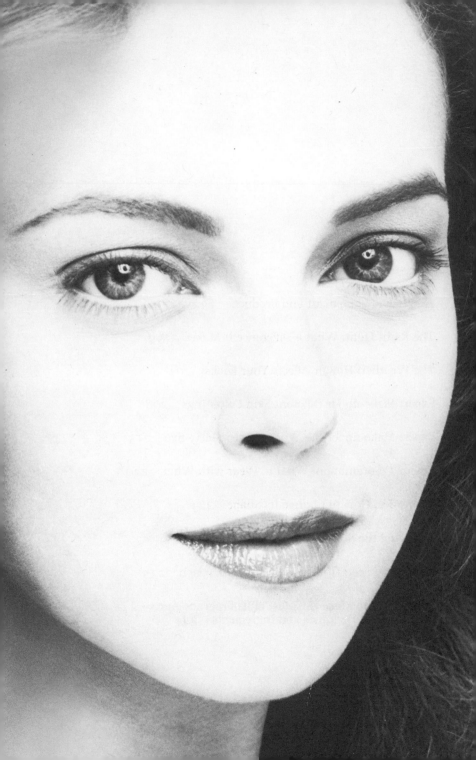

Introduction

It's incredible to think that for about 6,000 years women – and men – have used cosmetics. And, although the arts of make-up and hairdressing have come quite a long way since early Egyptian ladies painted their faces, anointed their bodies and spent so many hours achieving the dramatic effects we associate with legendary beauties like Queen Nefertiti and Cleopatra, the amazing thing is that the basic cosmetic items remain the same. For hair: shampoos, conditioners and colourants; for face: foundation, eyeshadow, kohl, cheek rouge, lip and nail colour from the herb henna; for skin: creams and oil for both face and body; and, of course, scent. Cleopatra, for instance, was known to bathe in asses' milk, which she believed softened and improved her skin – and even now many skin and bath products are called milks, although, of course, they don't necessarily contain real milk. These early cosmetics may have been crude in content, colour and texture, and there was obviously not so much choice, but the categories were identical.

The Chinese are thought to have been the first to experiment with make-up, then the Egyptians who probably learned about the art from travellers returning from China and who have left us much more positive evidence, owing to their habit of burying personal possessions with mummified bodies in tombs. The excavation of these tombs has enabled museums today to display ancient relics of once vital beauty routines: cosmetics pots, which still contained traces of ointments when discovered; toilet spoons; containers for kohl and sticks for its application; palettes, bowls and pestles for grinding and mixing cosmetic colours; polished metal mirrors; and, of course, the valuable perfume containers. Also, there were hair-care aids – combs, curling tongs, etc. The early Egyptians wore wigs – mostly black, but some red, blue and green – and they were probably the first to use henna. The Greeks of the same period used coloured powders (gold, white, red) to tint their natural hair; the Romans bleached with ashes of plants. There were punks among the Gauls – they dyed their hair bright red with goat's grease and ashes of beech timber – and the Anglo-Saxons coloured their hair green, orange and blue.

The desire to paint the face and body is one of the most primitive known to man, appearing throughout the ancient civilizations. The Greeks were responsible for popularizing whitened complexions, achieved, unfortunately, through the use of white lead (later called ceruse), which proceeded to ruin women's complexions through all the whims of fashion until the end of the 19th century. More favourably, they are sometimes credited with the invention of scent – in their mythology, Aphrodite is said to have been the brilliant innovator. Baths were considered important enough for the production of scented, softening water-additives.

For centuries it was the heads of state, their consorts and the ladies and gentlemen who surrounded them who were arbiters of beauty. Legendary beauties like Helen of Troy and the Queen of Sheba paved the way for Nero's Empress Poppaea, Catherine de' Medici, Lucretia Borgia, the Saxon Queen Matilda and Eleanor of Aquitaine, who all showed an intense interest in their appearance. Elizabeth I was fascinated by fashion news from abroad, wore scented gloves, bathed in scented waters and, like her rival across the border, Mary Queen of Scots, turned her hair up and back over pads or wire frames to give height in front. Royal marriages linked countries throughout Europe and helped spread new ideas.

In 19th-century England dandies like Beau Brummell outshone the ladies, and aristocratic female beauty dimmed into an era of Victorian disapproval – insipid and plain. Focus began to be transferred from royal and high-society to stage personalities – like Lola

Montez, Lillie Langtry and Sarah Bernhardt.

Interest in the beauty of royalty was rekindled by King Edward's Queen Alexandra, who when she was Princess of Wales revived the fashion for painted faces. Then American beauties like Consuelo Vanderbilt and Jennie Jerome captured public imagination with their wealth, beauty and marriages (to the Duke of Marlborough and Lord Randolph Churchill). Then came the 1914–18 war, after which nothing was the same.

The emancipation of women brought many changes in their appearance – they cut their hair, showed their ankles and expressed an individualism in their looks. The wide distribution of silent movies with stars like Theda Bara and Marion Davies created a real demand for cosmetics – to help women emulate them – and a mass interest in beauty that is still growing today.

The Second World War, however, brought an economy in everything – neat, practical hair styles, powder and lipstick, square shoulders and short skirts were the style of the forties – but the lean years during and after the War were relieved by dreams of looking like the screen goddesses of the time. Their influence was superseded by the fashion models, who were envied and copied.

Then the scene shifted once more and fashion encouraged a healthy, girl-next-door kind of naturalness which needed care if it was not to fall into the trap of looking pale and uninteresting.

Slowing up the ageing process has been a major source of concern throughout history; now much can be done to prolong youth by keeping the body fit – with regular exercise, proper diet and good beauty routines. We are lucky enough to live in an era when science brings help within the reach of all women. Researchers into the mechanism of the human body are constantly making new discoveries in the world of health and medicine, and often new beauty aids are a welcome spin-off.

This book aims to tell you how to make the most of yourself – for healthy hair and skin and the right amount of make-up will keep you looking good much longer.

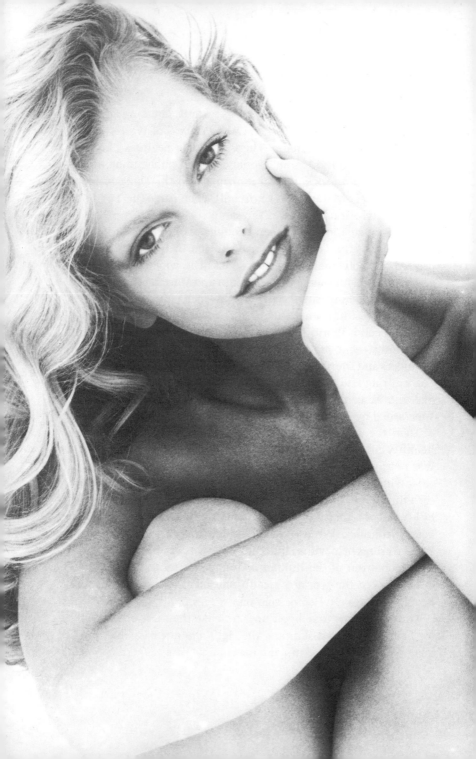

Skin:
What It Is and What It Does

Skin is a tissue covering the whole body – approximately one and a half square metres. It consists of areas called the *epidermis*, a visible surface layer with no blood-vessels; the *dermis*, full of collagen fibres, cells that store and release vital moisture, and nourishing blood-vessels; glands for lubrication (sebaceous) and for regulating body temperatures (sweat); and an important layer of fat that feeds the sebaceous glands and acts as a cushion between surface skin and muscle below. The epidermis, having no blood-vessels, will heal without trace. The dermis, on the other hand, if damaged, will result in scars: it is this layer, which is full of blood-vessels, that is affected by emotions and causes blushing and other changes in colour. Some people, for instance, turn white from panic or shock and this is caused by the draining-away of these blood-vessels; others turn green if they're feeling ill and this is a yellow bile from the liver coming to the surface through them. The glands function through the pores which are exit channels, visible to the eye and which, if the skin isn't cleaned properly, become clogged and form whiteheads or blackheads. It is the sebaceous glands which decide whether your skin is oily (they are over-active), dry (they are sluggish) or normal (they are functioning well). Beneath the scalp they will determine whether your hair is oily, dry or normal.

The depth and quality of your skin changes in different parts of the body. The scalp is densely populated with hair follicles fed by the sebaceous glands and needs to be kept scrupulously clean to avoid problems and encourage healthy hair. The face holds many

13

variations – the eye area is more transparent and delicate than anywhere else; the lips, mouth and inner nose are entirely different, being moist mucous membrane (likewise the vaginal area); the neck tends to be dry. Areas of the body normally covered by clothing retain their natural softness longer than limbs and extremities like hands and feet. The skin on palms and soles is the thickest and toughest of all. Then, there are armpits, which hold sweat-glands and contain more hair follicles; breasts, which have a transparent quality all their own; the genital area, which also has its own sweat-glands and hair follicles; and the gluteal fold of the buttocks. Hormones are essential to the satisfactory functioning of the body and play a vital part in the skin's activity: they stimulate pigment cells and regulate colour; they affect the production of sebum (so necessary to healthy hair); the secretion of the adrenal glands stimulates the sweat-glands; hormones control the breasts, which often change during the menstrual cycle and swell before menstruation, giving the skin a stretched translucent appearance and a feeling of discomfort from the extra liquid. Hormonal imbalance can cause enlarged pores, which sometimes leads to acne.

Nerves, too, are an important area. Contact is made through the skin, giving sensations such as tickling, touch, temperature changes, itching, pain, taste, smell and sexual arousal. Nerves vary in density in different areas of the body and vary from person to person – hence, one person may be ticklish in the ribs or soles of the feet, another not.

A good diet, exercise, sleep, fresh air and plenty of water are necessary if your skin is to look its best. On the other hand, it will react badly to emotional stress and tension and it will suffer from sun and wind if not protected. Deodorant-antiperspirants should be used sparingly or glands will cease to function properly; also avoid excessive washing and beware of unqualified 'beauticians' in fields like massage and hair removal.

Skin Types:
Which Is Yours?

Your ancestors and immediate parentage, through your genes, will have determined your skin colour and the bone structure which gives faces their characteristics. Your skin may be pale, olive, or black – with variations on all three – and your race descends from one of the ancient world's main four: Caucasian, Negro, Mongolian and Australian. All these probably developed from a single origin and have interbred over the centuries, so the distinctive features of skull shape, hair type and skin colour have diminished and probably rarely exist now in pure form. Whatever your race, skin is usually divided into four types: oily, dry, a combination of the two and balanced, with two subsidiary categories, sensitive and blemished. The word 'healthy' in relation to skin means smooth skin that glows with colour, is free of blemishes and is clean. This is the kind of skin you should have, and once you have discovered your skin type, provided you stick to a regular correct skin-treatment routine (and the wonderful thing about skin is that it does respond to care and can be improved), it is the kind of skin you can have.

Oily Skin
Oily skin comes from over-active sebaceous glands. It shines excessively, tends to break out and is the most likely candidate to suffer from acne. If you have oily skin you will probably also find you have enlarged pores and oily hair; you are also likely to be under twenty, after which hormones are more stable and skin

often undergoes a change for the better. It is to your advantage that oily skin develops fewer wrinkles and stays looking younger longer.

Blemished Skin
Blemished skin usually results from oily skin which has suffered from spots and acne and, in the worst cases, scarred permanently. It can also be the result of diseases like chicken-pox and measles.

Dry Skin
Dry skin tends to flake and has a matt texture with little or no shine. It is the result of dehydration – the sebaceous glands are sluggish, or the skin has been over-exposed to sun, wind and central heating. This type of skin rarely suffers from spots, and pores are hardly visible, but the condition doesn't improve with age and wrinkles will appear early.

Sensitive Skin
Sensitive skin is usually a consequence of dry skin, is often allergic to many cosmetics, tends to develop red patches from broken capillaries near the skin's surface and cannot be exposed to direct sunlight. Certain foods, alcoholic drinks, stress and emotional problems may also affect this type.

Combination Skin
Combination skin usually has a T-shaped panel of oiliness down the centre (across the forehead and down the middle and sides of the nose and mouth), with dry areas on cheeks and towards the hairline.

Balanced Skin
Balanced skin is what everyone would like to possess, but few do. The skin will appear fine-textured, smooth and well-coloured, will rarely break out and will retain its youthful quality well, although it will probably become drier after thirty.

Skin Care:
How to Treat Each Type

All skin will look better if a regular routine is followed, and the earlier it is started, the longer skin will keep its elasticity and youth. Teenagers need to learn that regular cleansing and moisturizing is as important as cleaning their teeth – and the sooner they learn about their skin type and its problems, the fewer they will suffer as they grow older.

Whatever your age, once you've discovered your skin type and chosen the products you are going to use, you must work out a routine that you know can become a lifetime habit. Just like a diet, it's no good attempting something that doesn't fit into your life-style. Cleanse, tone and moisturize are the three basic steps to remember.

All skin needs cleansing – to get rid of surface dirt and stale make-up and to loosen clogged pores. You may be a soap and water addict, and there is nothing better than this, provided the soap is mild, designed for your skin type and thoroughly rinsed off afterwards. Or there are cleansers which also need to be rinsed off with water. Creams, greases and oils are good for dissolving make-up, particularly those specially formulated for removing eye make-up (where soap and water may irritate), but you then need a freshener as well to remove excess grease. These oil-based products are almost always used for removing heavy or theatrical make-up. Oils are often recommended for sensitive dry skins, but even these types can be cleansed with soap and water if the correct strength is used.

All skins need a freshener. After cleansing, a certain amount of debris and oil will inevitably remain and must be removed. Fresheners, toners and astringents are all of the same family, containing more or less alcohol. They are alcohol-free for dry and sensitive skins, contain a small amount for combination or balanced skins, and more for oily skins, with the addition of anti-septic ingredients for blemished skins. They all aim to stimulate circulation and restore the acid mantle which may have become unbalanced in the cleansing process.

All skins need moisturizing. Natural moisture evaporates and needs containing in even the oiliest skin. Moisturizers form a film over the skin's surface, holding in the natural moisture and providing a smooth base for make-up or a protective barrier between the skin and the environment. There are lightweight, medium and heavier types of moisturizer – the richer ones being needed as the skin grows older, or if they are going to be used without the added protection of foundation.

Specialized Care for Oily Skin
Oily skin with its tendency to shine and break out needs the most efficient deep cleansing. It's a good idea to use a cleanser formulated especially for this skin type, and since it may need cleansing midday as well as night and morning, choose one that's effective but not harsh. Follow with an astringent to remove any last traces of oil, but avoid the eye area. Oily skins need moisturizing too, to help the skin retain its natural moisture and stop it evaporating too fast. A lightweight moisturizer that leaves a matt surface on the skin is the one to look for, and if you find it too rich for daytime use, try using it only at night.

Even if oily skin persists as you get older, you will need eye and throat creams for those areas to combat wrinkles.

The use of a cleansing mask twice a week will help clear clogged pores, remove dead cells and refine the skin's texture.

Specialized Care for Blemished Skin
Basic care is the same as for oily skin, with the addition of medicated lotions to fight the bacteria that are causing problems. If the condition is severe, professional advice should be sought from a trained beautician, who may recommend medical help from your doctor or a dermatologist.

Specialized Care for Dry Skin
To keep dry skin at its delicate best, give it a good gentle cleansing night and morning. Night cleansing is very important since you have a day's accumulation of dirt and make-up to remove. A mild soap-and-water rinseable cleanser or cleansing cream is good for dry skin. Follow this with a light, non-alcoholic freshener – avoid anything called an astringent. A rich moisturizer should be used during the day, a nourishing cream at night, with specialized creams for eyes and throat.

A weekly exfoliating treatment will help to reduce flakiness, and a stimulating mask will encourage the glands to produce more natural lubricants.

Specialized Care for Sensitive Skin
Basic care is the same as for dry skin, with special attention to allergies. Look for sun-care and other products in hypoallergenic ranges. Most large cosmetic companies put their products through extensive allergy tests before putting them on the market, but those marked hypoallergenic are further tested for less common allergies.

Specialized Care for Combination Skin
Combination skin consists of dry and oily patches which need separate care. It is caused by the natural concentration of glands being heavier in some parts of the face than in others – normally in a T-shaped area across the forehead and down the nose. It is often too expensive to have different products for each area, so the

answer is to use mild soap and water, or a cleanser that is not too abrasive for the dry areas but will clean the oily areas too. A mild toner, either non-alcoholic or with a small amount which can be diluted with water for the dry patches, is useful to remove excess grease and stimulate the circulation. Then, a medium-rich moisturizer is essential, concentrating on the dry parts, plus a special cream for eye area and neck. A clearing mask once a week down the centre panel will make all the difference to the balance of the skin.

Specialized Care for Balanced Skin

Basic care is the same as for dry skin, as even the best-behaved has a tendency to dry out as it grows older. To keep it at its best, a good cleanse, tone and moisturize routine is essential, and a weekly stimulating-mask treatment will encourage it to keep up the good work.

All skin types will benefit from an occasional visit to a beauty salon for a deep-cleanse treatment. The professional beautician will cleanse the skin, perhaps using the latest electronic equipment and paying attention to blackheads and whiteheads; stimulate the circulation with light massage using fingers or mechanical aids; and choose a good mask to help the particular condition of your skin. It is a good idea to make your appointment when you know you needn't wear make-up for a good twelve or, even better, twenty-four hours afterwards. This gives the skin time to breathe and benefit from the treatment it has received. Another good idea is to change the products you use occasionally. Just as your body benefits from a change of diet from time to time, so does your skin. However, ranges are formulated to work together, i.e. the ingredients of cleanser, moisturizer and toner that one company makes are designed to complement each other, so your skin is more likely to gain maximum benefit from them together than if you mix the different brands; also, they need to be used for several months or until they need replacing, if they are to do the job for which they were intended.

Steve Svensson

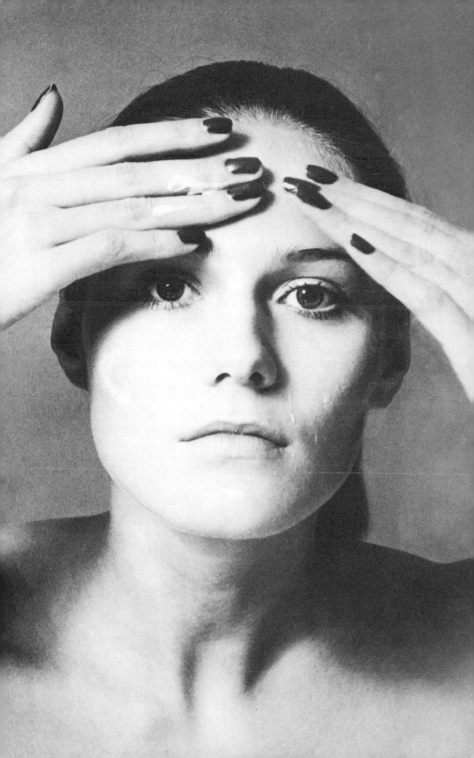

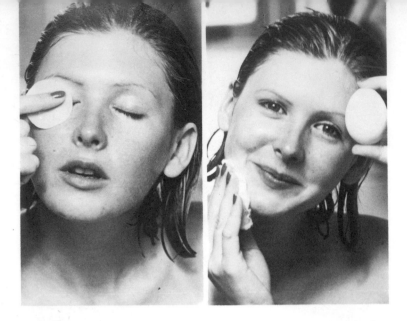

Cleansing pads *are good for removing mascara and stubborn eye make-up*

Toners and astringents *are after-cleansing agents for skin tightening and brightening*

Soap and water *give an unbeatable clean feeling; pure soaps won't dry or irritate the face*

Masks *strip off city grime, unclog pores and let the skin breathe*

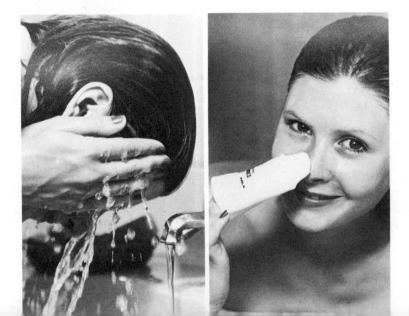

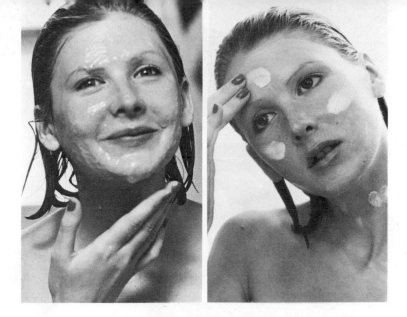

Gels *wake up sluggish skin and get it glowing*
Moisturizers *should be part of every skin's beauty routine morning and night*
Foams *are fluffy cleansers that whip on quickly*
All-in-ones *are multipurpose – a cleanser that's also a face-wash or shampoo; a moisturizer that works for face, legs and hands; a colour to highlight and blush*

Steve Svensson

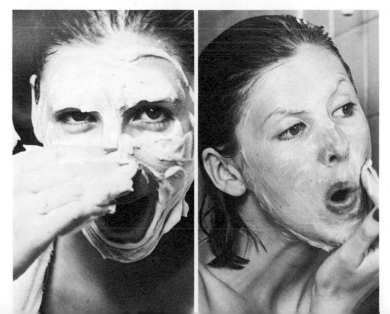

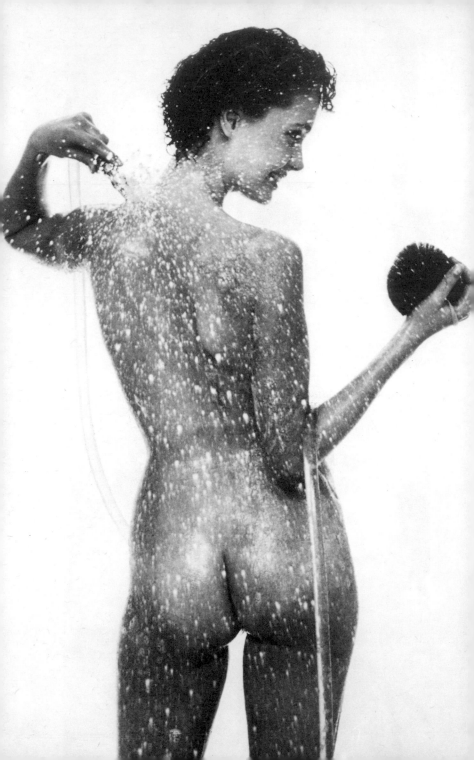

Cleansing the Body:
Baths and Showers

There is no question about it, all-over beauty begins in the bathroom. Cleansing the body is just as important as cleansing the face, and baths (or showers) are the only way to keep it clean and fresh. Most body odours, if allowed free access to fresh air, will evaporate quickly, and the smell, if any, will be quite pleasant. But, our civilization demands that our bodies are clothed 95 per cent of the time, and clothes (particularly those made of synthetic fibres) trap body moisture which quickly forms bacteria. It is the bacteria, not the sweat, that smell and become unpleasant. Deodorants are one way to attack the problem, but regular washing goes a long way towards solving it.

The bathroom itself should be a most relaxing and comfortable room – not something shoved into the only space available, with no heat, cold linoleum and draughty windows. In America many people have their make-up table and hair accessories in the bathroom too, thus making it a beauty room rather than merely functional. This sensible idea, along with proper lighting surrounding good mirrors, is gradually being adopted in Europe, and even existing cheerless bathrooms can be improved now there are wall-heaters, washable wall coverings and carpets, and now that draughts can be excluded. Mirrors are pretty (and an essential aid to beauty), certain plants thrive in the steamy atmosphere of a bathroom and well-placed lighting does much to ease pressure and tension. Take a new look at your bathroom and see what can be improved, then start discovering the pleasures of the bath.

Never try to get into a bath that is too hot, or stay in a hot bath too long. It is enervating and draws away too much of the body's natural moisture and oil, leaving you exhausted, your skin dry and often wrinkled.

A warm bath is best (not over 100°F or 38°C) as a general rule. A lukewarm bath is refreshing on very hot days (much more so than a cold dip, which has only a temporary effect) and a tepid one is a good pick-up at any time. Cold baths are traditionally bracing and cold water is easiest to brave under a shower – this is most stimulating, and if you can get really strong pressure from the water, it will not only improve circulation but exercise muscles too.

If your only object is to clean your body, then all you need is soap and water and something to dry it – sunshine or a towel. Possibly, if you are short of time, this is the sort of bath you need occasionally, but it takes no more time to add a moisturizing oil while it is running, and to use a fragrant soap. However, cleansing is not the only function of baths. Baths can relax the mind and muscles, soften and nourish the skin, stimulate the circulation, invigorate the mind and clear the head – which you choose usually depends on the time of day and the amount of time you can allow yourself, plus a thought for your general state of health.

First thing in the morning you need a good start to the day – it may be a *soothing transition* from sleep, in which case fragrant oils are a good idea, and an unhurried soak in warm water. Or, you may need a *brisk wake-up* and toner for relaxed muscles, so try a citrus or pine-scented essence in lukewarm water. Or, if your system needs a *real shock* to get it started, smooth over a body shampoo, rinse off under the shower with warm water, then turn the tap sharply to cold.

After a rough day, you need at least ten minutes for a *quiet bath* (remember to take the telephone off the hook, put on some gentle music and make sure you are not disturbed). This will revitalize you for the evening, and if you choose a hot bath, try and take a cool rinse afterwards for extra energy. A home-made infusion of herbs specially mixed for their soothing, calming, moisturizing properties is excellent at this time. Use dried herbs – grow your own and dry them, or buy them ready-dried. Then put your mixture in a muslin bag and tie it firmly to the hot tap so the water runs through it. Your *herbal bath* should include flowers as well as leaves (picked from roses, camomiles or lavender, elders or lemon-trees), pine-needles and any herbs you discover and like, such as fennel, thyme, rosemary, sage and peppermint. For instance, try a blackberry bath as a tonic for your skin ... make a strong infusion and use it for two or three nights running. A pine bath to refresh ... boil pine-needles for half an hour and allow them to steep overnight; strain and use a cupful in each bath. A lemon bath to invigorate ... add slices to a lemon-scented bath oil and use slices to rub over your skin. An elder bath for soothing ... in infusion form. A lavender bath for pleasure ... dried lavender flowers mixed with a little dried mint and rosemary. Alternatively, choose one of the ready-mixed herbal concoctions available or the delicious products which include herbs in the ingredients. Last thing before bed, a *lazy warm bath* encourages sleep – it should be redolent of sweet-smelling flowers, with moisturizing foam or milk. Pat yourself dry afterwards – don't rub vigorously and don't take your bath too soon after a meal. There are variations to try at any time:

The country bath. Everyone knows what a day in the country does for morale and beauty. A country-smelling bath allows you to dream yourself into the same state. Without taking a step you can conjure up fields of flowers, old-fashioned herb gardens, a glade of bluebells or hedgerow of honeysuckle, wild roses and moss. Try gels that blend extracts of marigold and pine-needles, soften the water and cleanse the body ... essences that soften and scent the water ... oils that soften, cleanse and nourish the skin.

A flowery bath. There's nothing more delightful than to receive a beautiful bouquet of flowers. Almost as good, but better for your skin, is a fragrantly flowery bath. Choose a milk bath with the bouquet of honeysuckle, rose and spices – and use talcum powder, body cream and deodorant in matching fragrance to help the scent linger ... a foam bath or oil to soften or to colour your bath a delicious sea-blue or green.

A sea-water bath, if you long for that breezy tang of a holiday. There are lots of bath additives using sea algae, which contain all the minerals of sea water that help draw toxic substances from the body and ease rheumatic complaints, aching joints and muscles.

As with everything else, you need the right equipment to get the most out of your bath: a rough-textured loofah, perfect for removing dead skin and leaving the body tingling; a sponge for soaping your skin (when it becomes clogged with soap, steep overnight in vinegar to freshen it); nail-brush and body brush – choose them with stiff, natural bristles; pumice-stone for rubbing away rough skin on heels, soles of the feet and elbows; flannel or bath mitt made of cotton towelling for rubbing on soap (make sure you launder them frequently or they'll harden with the soap residue).

After your bath your skin is at its most receptive – this is the moment, when it is completely dry, to use a deodorant, lots of moisturizing body lotion, a splash of cologne and talcum powder; if your finger- or toenails need cutting, they are soft and pliant after a bath, and it is a good moment to massage cuticles with a nourishing cream.

Barry Lategan

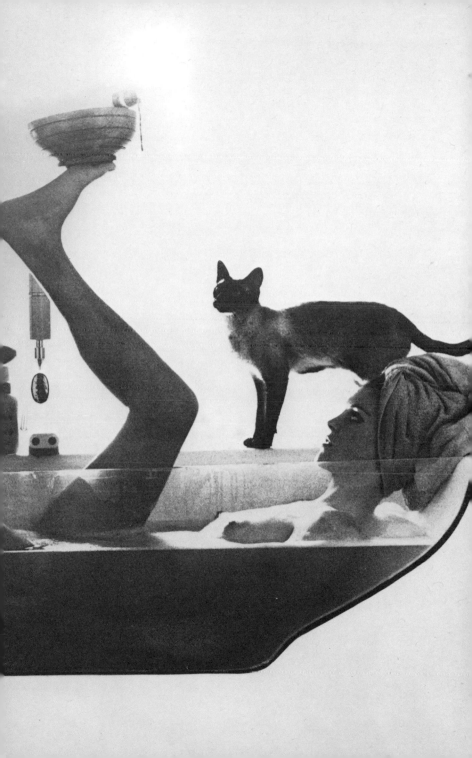

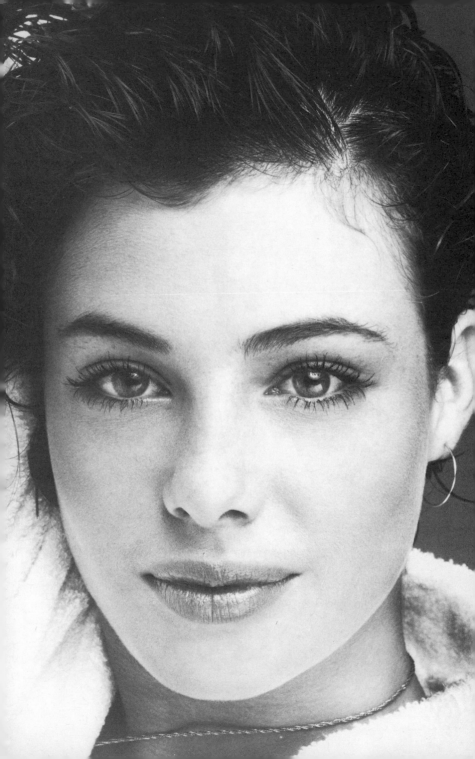

Beauty Products:
What Does What Do to Your Face?

Basic beauty kit for taking proper care of the skin on your face should include cleanser, eye make-up remover, toner, moisturizer, plus (depending on your age and individual needs) night cream, eye cream, throat cream and various masks.

Cleansers. There are foam cleansers, gel cleansers, cream cleansers, milky cleansers, cleansing oils and, of course, the original soap and water routine. (The modern cleansing bar is totally non-alkaline and contains no soap of any kind. It can be used in any kind of water, hard or soft. It contains an emulsifying agent similar to that used in a cleansing cream, plus solidifying agents that turn the cream into a bar.) Which you use is a matter of personal preference, but the point of cleansing your skin is to clean it. New-born babies are bathed and cleaned with oils; children and teenagers, even before starting to use make-up, should learn to clean their face, not just to remove visible food or dirt but all over, to clear it of grime accumulated during the day which, if allowed to become ingrained, will cause spots and blackheads. Later it becomes obvious that stale make-up needs removing thoroughly and the skin needs frequent cleansing.

Special eye make-up removers. These become necessary as more and more people want water- or smudge-proof make-up. This make-up clings to the face and so becomes more difficult to remove, and ordinary cleansers, particularly soap and water, have a tendency to irritate the eyes. There are creams, oils and liquids to choose from – also boxes of pads saturated with a cleanser which are neat and easy to use.

Toners. Either an alcohol-free freshener, a mild toner or an astringent is necessary to remove any traces of cleanser, to close the pores and generally brighten up the skin's texture before the application of moisturizer.

Moisturizers. These help to replace the natural moisture lost through evaporation and act as a barrier protecting the skin from air pollution or as a preparatory base for foundation, making it easier to blend in and look natural.

Night creams. These are a richer form of moisturizer containing extra lubricants to help combat wrinkles and ageing. Young people and sufferers from oily skin often find a day-time moisturizer sufficient for night-time use.

Eye creams and throat creams are nourishing creams specially formulated to feed the skin in those areas. They are usually used at night, although the newer formulations are less and less greasy and are often recommended for day-time use too.

Masks can cleanse, revitalize, condition, stimulate or exfoliate. They are applied all over the face, avoiding the eye area and mouth, left to dry for a certain time and then either rinsed or peeled off. They are always included in a professional facial when the type will be decided for you, but for home use be sure you buy the variety you want.

Cleansing masks have a deep-down action, helping to free clogged pores, loosen blackheads, remove surface dirt and clear dead cells.

Revitalizing masks often provide the quick pick-up your face needs before going out for the evening; they can be applied before a bath and will have done their job by the time you are out and dry – in about 10–15 minutes.

Conditioning masks do just that. They give your face an occasional deep treat and are particularly good if you don't use a night cream, as they provide the extra nourishment your skin needs.

Stimulating masks purify the skin and activate circulation, pumping more oxygen to the surface and leaving the blood-vessels

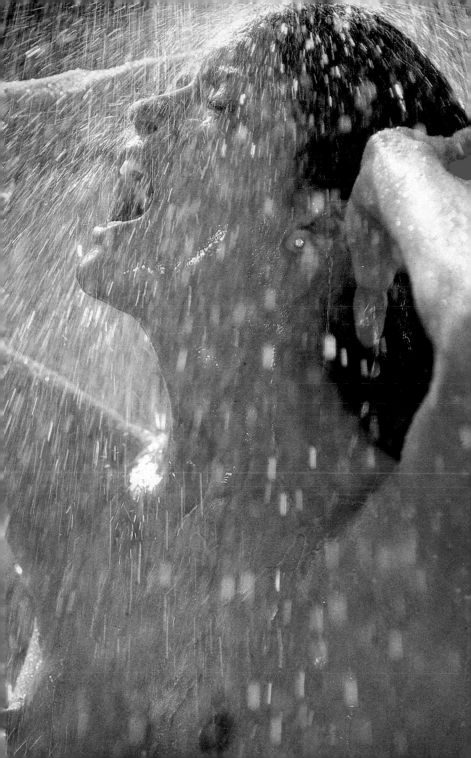

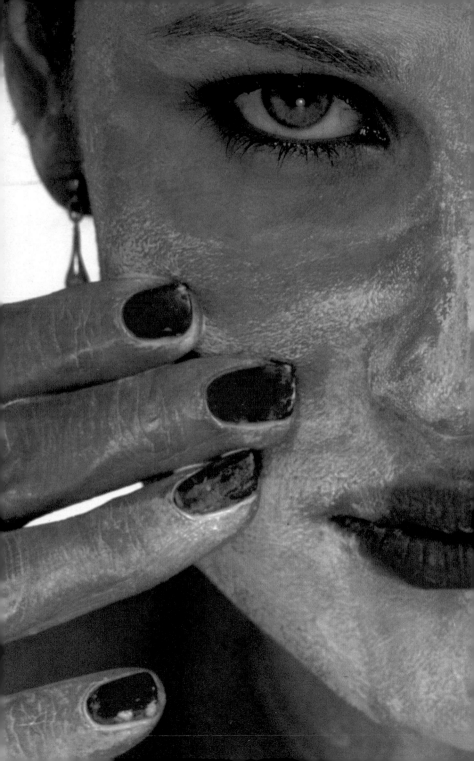

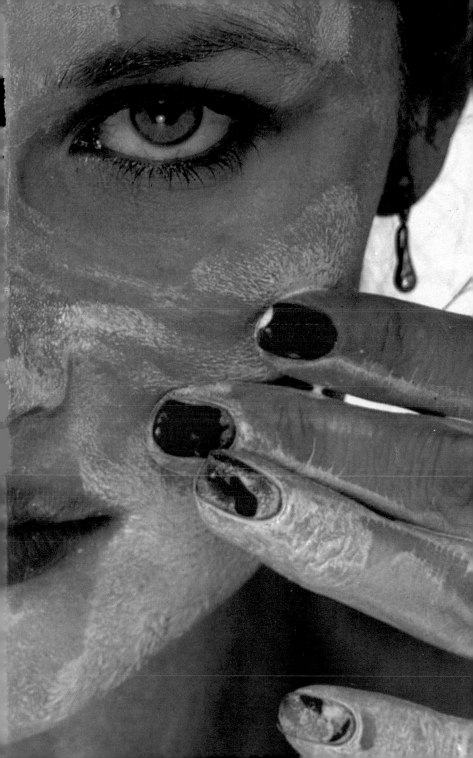

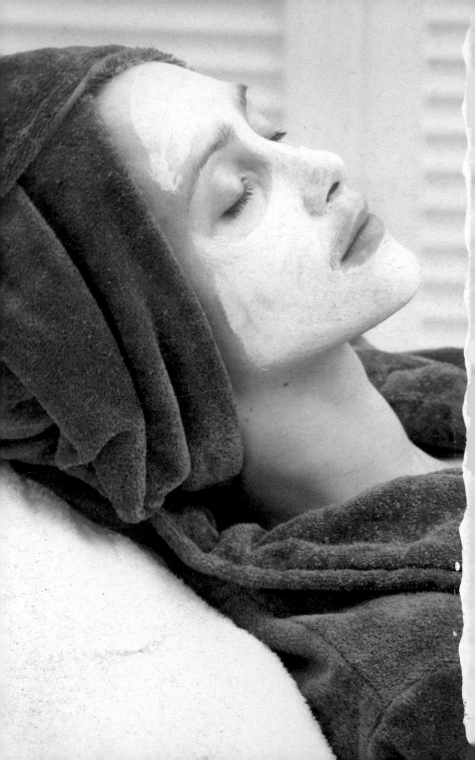

enlarged so that the skin will look pink when it's removed. This increased circulation will improve the skin's colour and texture.

Exfoliating masks are designed especially for the removal of dead cells from the surface of the skin and are really a gentle form of peeling (only practised to get rid of lines, soften scars and remove blemishes, and only done by qualified specialists). The dead cells are what often give the skin a grey look or blotchy tone, and the use of an exfoliating mask will brighten the appearance and smooth the texture.

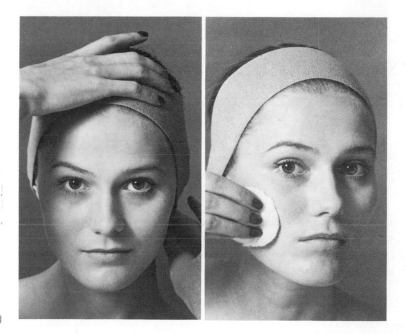

Step-by-Step Facial
I. Put a headband or tie a scarf around your hairline to keep hair out of face and lotions out of hair. 2. Apply a gentle cleanser with a cotton-wool pad. To do this the professional way, use motions that 'cut across'

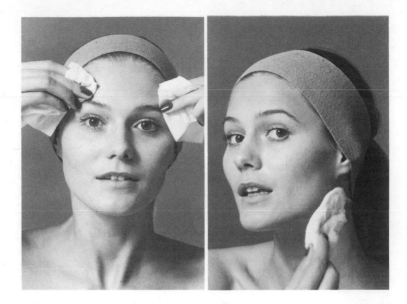

skin lines and wrinkles. Use up and down strokes on forehead, horizontal movements above lips and on chin, and for the eye area, a motion that starts at cheek, comes towards nose and up across brows. These movements help to discourage more wrinkles and should be used both when applying and when removing skin-care products. **3.** *Tissue off the cleanser, making sure to use the motions described.* **4.** *Apply a toner to remove last traces of cleanser and tighten pores slightly. You are now ready for a mask.* **5.** *(opposite) Put on a light moisturizer, dotting it on forehead, cheeks and chin, then blending it in with fingertips. Again use the motions described.* **6.** *Rinse skin with clear luke-warm water, then apply mask. Leave on for prescribed time and relax.* **7.** *To make the most of your rest, apply cotton-wool pads soaked in skin tonic to your eyes for a soothing, cool feeling.* **8.** *Remove mask and blot – do not rub face with a towel. Finish off with a thin film of moisturizer.*

William Connors

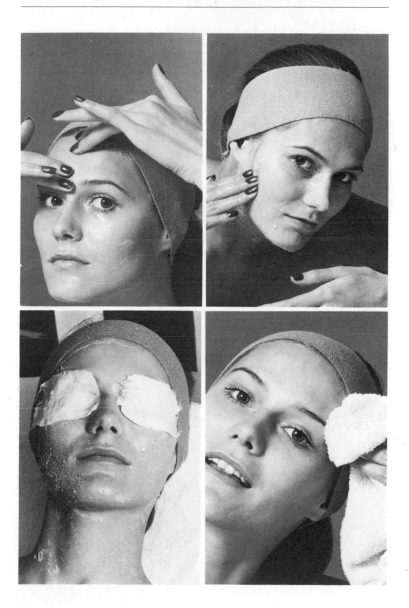

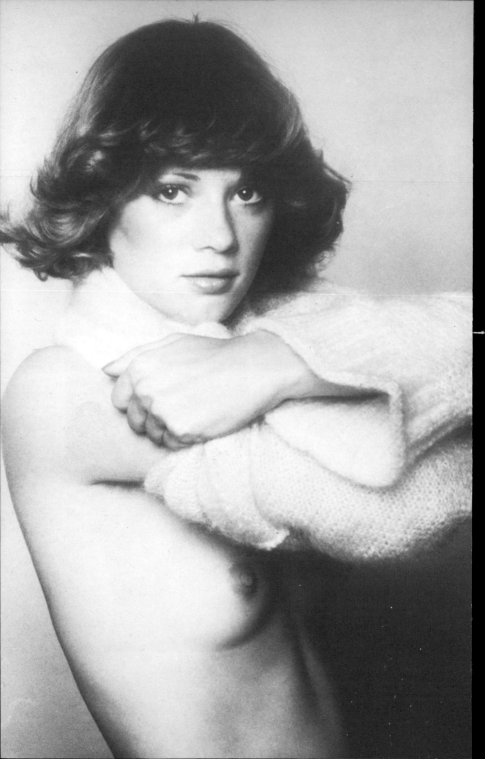

Age:
What Happens When?

Most of us are lucky and were born whole. We contain all the proper organs (intestines, glands, veins, blood and so on), we have features and limbs and hair where they should be and our skin is unblemished. In fact we have everything intended for the perfect human being – and it's all in good working order. But, as we grow older, the body becomes used and abused, and changes take place. Skin, in particular, goes through phases and is susceptible to various problems at these times. Even babies may suffer early from rashes, allergies and problems related to their skin type which continue through childhood.

Teens

Puberty causes a tremendous upheaval in the body, with hormonal activity affecting every gland and consequently the skin. Skin, which until now may have behaved beautifully, suddenly starts playing up and erupting into *acne*. This is the result of hormones stimulating the oil glands into over-production of oil, which gets clogged in the pores. This is so prevalent among adolescents – girls and boys – that it is often dismissed as something they must just endure until it goes away. But, treatment is available, and if the course is followed properly, the skin condition will certainly improve and, depending on its severity, may disappear. Another problem connected with this hormonal activity is that the *hair* follicles all over the body are stimulated into growth and it sometimes appears in unwanted places – above the upper lip and on the sides of the face, for instance. However, once the body has settled into its new pattern, this facial hair often falls out and doesn't return; if it is dark and very obvious it can be lightened with a special facial hair bleach, but more serious forms of removal should be left for several years.

Enlarged pores, sometimes a symptom of oily skin, sometimes resulting from acne, but caused by excess oil clogging and then stretching the pores, are also a sign of adolescence. They don't disappear, so scrupulous cleansing to prevent their arrival is the answer. Another condition – seen by some as a problem, by others as an attractive asset – is freckles. These often go hand in hand with the pale translucent skin possessed by natural red-heads and are actually cells containing extra quantities of melanin (a dark pigment stimulated by sunlight into turning brown) grouped together in the skin. They will increase in the sunshine, but often fade in the winter months and can only temporarily be removed. However, a good sun block (see p. 65) will help to curtail their numbers.

Twenties

This is when your skin should look its best – it has been through the upheaval of adolescence and is not yet on the road to decline, although it will show signs of ageing in the late twenties if care is not taken. In fact most problems that appear now are caused by lack of care in the teens. Neglect during those years, and sometimes the use of cosmetics designed for a more mature skin (borrowed from mother perhaps, or lent with the best intentions) can result in *acne* appearing now. Or it can be the result of going on the Pill.

If *freckles* or *brown spots* appear at this stage and seem to be the variety that don't fade in winter, they aren't natural and are probably caused by over-exposure to the sun, which will also hasten the ageing process later on. These blemishes are removable by a dermatologist, but after treatment great care should be taken not to expose the skin to the sun.

Skin allergies usually become apparent in the twenties – when

38

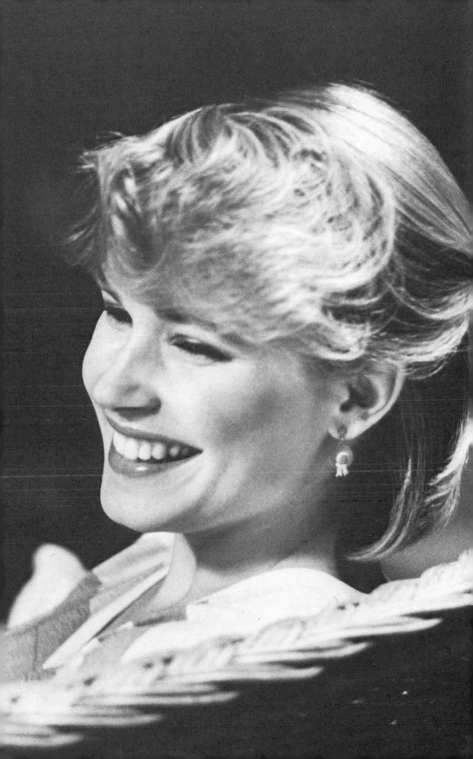

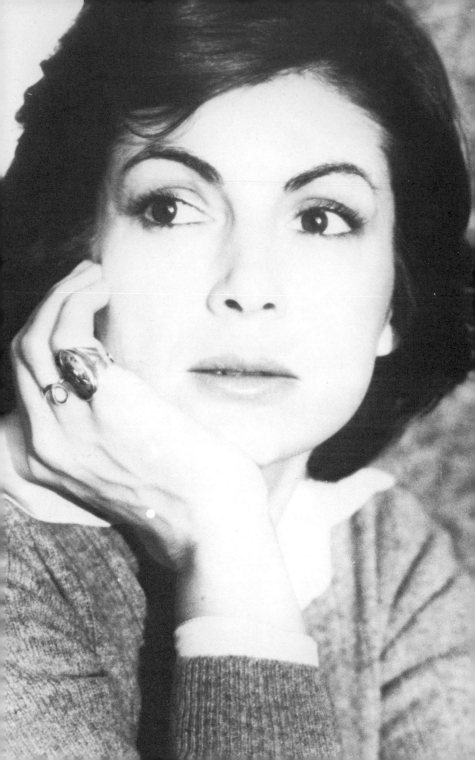

women have started working in offices or factories or running their own homes and thus handle industrial equipment and office machinery or have contact with detergents, insecticides and so on. They often continue to use many different cosmetics and fragrances; they may travel more, experimenting with foreign foods. Any of these may cause an allergic reaction. The way to treat an allergy is to isolate it, then protect yourself as much as possible. This may involve a series of allergy tests to discover the cause.

Thirties

This is the time to guard against skin drying out and causing premature ageing. Change your skin-care routine to one formulated for more mature skins and watch out for a variety of acne called *dry skin acne*. This is thought to be caused by a special kind of oil, containing quantities of fatty acids, irritating the pores. Dry skin acne takes the form of blackheads and whiteheads, mostly on the chin and jaw-line. Women who have had dry skin all their lives will probably start noticing lines – fine ones, but lines all the same – and *bags* may appear under the eyes, removable only by cosmetic surgery, although, if caused by fluid from allergy or sinus problems, antihistamines can sometimes prevent the formation of these pouches.

Broken blood vessels, due to skin damage from pregnancy, excess alcohol, high blood pressure or a blow to the skin, may begin to show on the cheeks and around the nose as small red lines. These can usually be treated by a doctor.

Forties

The skin is beginning to lose its tone and strength – it finds it difficult to support the pores, and they start becoming more visible and may become *enlarged*. Masks and astringents will help temporarily. Another variety of acne – *acne rosacea* – often appears during the forties. Its exact cause is not known, although stress, alcohol, spicy foods and extremes of hot and cold are known to aggravate the condition. It has a flushed appearance with blackheads and small pustules and can be treated by a dermatologist. *Psoriasis* also, although it can occur at any age, is most likely to appear now, its round red patches flecked with silvery scales showing first on elbows and knees. It is very difficult to cure.

Fifties and Onwards

The skin must begin to show its age however well it's been looked-after. It is no longer receiving sufficient support and elasticity from the protein fibres, and the fatty deposits beneath the skin are disappearing, leaving it loose and flabby. Lines deepen into *wrinkles*, the skin dries and the *drying skin* itself becomes a problem, sometimes with painful side-effects like itching, a slowness to heal and a tendency to become infected. Little clusters of *red lines* called *spider angiomata* may appear, as may *brown spots*. Deterioration in skin colour is often due to poor circulation and can be improved by massage and exercise. Most serious of all, this is the time when *skin cancer* usually appears. Of the four basic types, *solar keratoses*, which manifests itself in rough red patches, is the mildest. It is most commonly found in people who have sunbathed too much and for too long, people involved in outdoor sports or who lead outdoor lives. It can be treated but if left too long can develop into the more serious *squamous cell carcinoma*, a thicker, rougher growth. Both these types usually show first on the face – which is also usually the first area to be affected by a persistent sore that doesn't heal called *basal cell carcinoma*. All three types are treatable, but the last two may leave some scarring. The last type, and fortunately the least common, as it is by far the most serious, is *malignant melanoma*. The first sign is a deeply pigmented area on the skin coloured brown, black or even dark blue, which acts as a warning that there is a growth. A lump which changes colour or size when exposed to the sun may also indicate this type of cancer and should be checked immediately. The treatment is to remove the growth and a large area of the skin which surrounds it.

Arthur Elgort

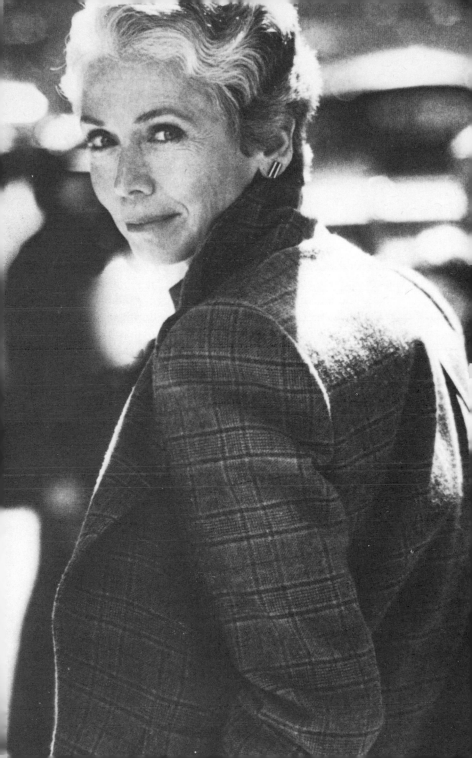

An A–Z of Common Skin Problems

Acne

Treatment for acne has developed tremendously in recent years. The condition is caused by over-activity of the sebaceous glands, which causes too much oil to flow, thus clogging and irritating the pores. Its occurrence is easily understandable during the hormonal changes undergone in adolescence; less easy to understand are the types of acne that flare up later. These vary with the age at which they appear. It is now thought that an exaggerated emphasis has been put on the connection between foods, such as chocolate, and acne and that the condition is not usually caused by dirt.

Teenage acne is synonymous with adolescence and causes much distress. Modern treatment discourages abrasive and over-zealous cleaning as this is thought to over-stimulate the oil glands into renewed activity. Gentle washing in conjunction with a special lotion has a better long-term effect. Low doses of the antibiotic oxytetracycline are frequently prescribed by doctors and dermatologists and are effective in alleviating severe acne. So too is a treatment involving retinoic acid. This works by loosening and softening the hardened keratin which is plugging the pores and causing the acne. Teenage acne should clear by the age of twenty-one, but if it hasn't it's likely to go on well into the thirties.

Acne which appears during the twenties is sometimes caused by birth-control pills, neglect of the skin during the teenage years or by the use of rich cosmetics designed for a more mature skin and inadequate cleansing.

Stress acne is likely to occur in the thirties; it appears suddenly in the form of large painful cysts with no accompanying blackheads, pustules or oily skin. Women under stress can, overnight, find their normally clear skin in trouble. One treatment is to inject the cyst with cortisone.

Dry skin acne is also common at this age – contradicting the idea that acne and oily skin are linked. This kind of acne is caused by a specific kind of oil, thought to contain large amounts of fatty acids, which irritates the pores until they erupt, usually into blackheads and whiteheads around the chin and jaw-line. This is normally treated with a low dose of tetracycline.

Acne rosacea is most likely to attack in the forties – arriving with a rosy flush and quickly followed by blackheads and small pustules. Its exact cause isn't known, but alcohol, spicy foods, stress and tension, extreme heat or intense cold are thought to aggravate the condition. Low doses of tetracycline will suppress the problem and a sulphur lotion is often helpful.

Extreme symptoms – excessively oily skin, facial hair, large quantities of cysts, for instance – indicate a real hormonal disorder, and dermatologists will often refer these cases to specialists to determine the cause before treating the problem further.

Allergies
One widespread cause of skin distress is allergic reaction. If you break out in spots or rashes, the cause may be something you have eaten or just touched; this is known as contact allergy. *Where* the outbreak occurs is often a clue to the problem – with the common nickel allergy, for instance, a reaction may appear just where a belt buckle or jeans fastener touched the skin. Skin allergies often become apparent in the twenties – after a few years in an office, factory or running a home and being in contact with office equipment, industrial machinery or everyday products like detergents. And by this time some women have developed an allergy to certain cosmetics – nail-polish is a well-known example,

showing not around the fingers, but where they touch the face (around the eyes, lips, etc.). As a rule modern cosmetics are very safe to use, being stringently tested before they are put on the market and using formulae which avoid any known irritants. To treat an allergy, the cause must be identified, and if it's not quickly obvious, this may entail a series of tests prescribed by a dermatologist, usually done in groups of patches on the back.

Athlete's Foot

This is a kind of ringworm that thrives in warm damp areas – most commonly found between toes and on the soles of the feet, occasionally between fingers. It is an infection picked up from going barefoot in communal areas, when enough care hasn't been taken to dry the feet after being immersed in water, or when they have sweated into socks that are left unchanged. The skin looks white and opaque, can itch and forms thick blisters which peel.

Bags

Under-eye bags are often hereditary, but during the thirties they can appear as a result of severe allergy or sinus problems where fluid is emptied into the area; this stretches the delicate skin, which loses its ability to spring back and so sags. The only real treatment for these pouches is cosmetic surgery.

Blackheads

Blackheads are not coloured by dirt but by melanin, the substance that makes skin and hair the colour they are. The darker your skin, the blacker they will be (very fair people are less prone to them as their skins are usually drier as well). They should not be prodded or poked as this is likely to cause enlargement and infection. Gentle, thorough cleansing softens the plug, bringing it to the surface and making it easy to rinse away; persistent blackheads should be treated by a trained beautician.

Blushing
This is a common physical sign of what's going on emotionally in the head – normally embarrassment, shame or anger. Some people only suffer on the face; with others the face remains pale while the chest starts to go red and the blush creeps up the neck. It is frustrating, and nothing has yet been discovered to control it – *you* certainly can't.

Blotchy Skin
If this only appears occasionally on the face, neck or chest it is probably an emotional blush, but if it is more widespread and permanent it is probably due to bad circulation. Massage and exercise will probably help.

Brown Spots
Brown spots appear on sun-abused skin in early life – the twenties – and are a normal part of skin ageing as you grow older. There are creams which can fade them and they can be removed without scarring by a dermatologist.

Cellulite
This is sometimes called *peau d'orange* because the skin over the affected area has the crinkly appearance of orange peel. The condition is caused by deposits of stubborn fat and excess water-retention accumulating beneath the skin, most likely on thighs, hips, buttocks and the upper arms. It affects thin as well as fat people and is very difficult to dislodge permanently. Massage alone is seldom very helpful as it often just moves the problem from one area to another. Breaking up and dissolving the deposits by a combination of exercise, diet and specialized salon treatment is the only effective way to reduce it, while healthy eating and proper exercise from an early age are the best ways to avoid it. Keeping a check on fluid-retention by eating foods that contain potassium

(which helps excrete excess salt) and drinking lots of good mineral water is also a good idea.

Corns
There are hard corns and soft corns – hard ones usually appear on joints, soft ones between toes – which grow on feet as a warning against ill-fitting shoes. Pressure causes a hardening of the skin which, if left unrelieved (special felt circles are widely available for this), will form a horny corn with the apex pointing inwards. Further pressure put on this apex causes intense pain. Corns should be treated by a chiropodist – amateur cutting and scraping can result in infection.

Cysts
These appear as solid little lumps either under the skin, usually the result of blocked sweat-glands, or in the ovaries where, if not detected and removed, they can grow to enormous sizes. There is a variety called a ganglion which usually appears near joints, e.g. on the hands near the wrists. These are filled with a clear jelly-like substance and can easily be removed surgically.

Dermatitis or Eczema
This is an inflammation of the skin that can appear anywhere on the body; it is red and often produces a mass of small blister-like bumps or dry scaly skin. There are many variations. The usual cause is an external irritant, i.e. an allergy to something in the sufferer's daily life, but nerves and emotions are also closely connected.

Enlarged Pores
These are caused by a permanent stretching of pores clogged by excess oil and often result from acne – even the mildest attack. Like anything else that is stretched beyond its capacity to spring back, once a pore becomes enlarged it is impossible to reduce it.

Prevention by careful cleansing and immediate attention to any problem is essential.

Facial Hair
This is often a teenage problem resulting from the hormonal changes occurring in the body and is most often seen around the upper lip and along the sides of the face. Once the hormones have settled down, this hair often falls out, never to return, but if it is dark and unsightly it can safely be lightened with a specifically formulated bleach. More drastic forms of removal such as electrolysis or waxing should be left until the problem appears to have become permanent at the end of adolescence.

Flabby Skin
This can appear in the young as a result of lack of exercise and poor diet and can be tightened up with a course of regular exercises and massage if these steps are taken soon enough. Flabby skin is also often the result of sudden weight-loss through illness or a too drastic diet and a return to fitness will depend on age and the amount of elasticity remaining in the skin.

Freckles
Certain people – often red-heads – are born with skin prone to freckles, which are groups of cells in the skin containing above-normal amounts of the dark pigment called melanin. They will fade in the winter, increase in the summer, can be reduced with a mild chemical peeling, but will return on re-exposure to sunlight. They are often very attractive, but if the possessor wants to keep them to a minimum, the use of a sun block (see p. 65) is essential in spring and summer. Freckles that appear later in life are called Brown Spots (see p. 47).

Frostbite
This is caused by exposure to intense cold and the stoppage of the

blood flow in vessels close to the skin's surface. The affected area – most often nose, fingers, toes or ears – becomes white, hard and numb and, if not treated fast, will cause permanent damage to the skin. The best treatment is to restore circulation with very gentle warmth such as bathing in cool water, although the area will become painfully inflamed and may produce rupturing blisters. Minor frostbite can be prevented by wearing enough suitable warm loose-fitting clothes to keep circulation going and, if skiing, for instance, in very cold conditions, frequently checking any exposed areas on yourself or your companions.

Lines
These are usually noticed around the eye area in the thirties and can come from allergies or sinus problems, particularly in conjunction with under-eye bags, or from worry or shock. Keeping the area well-moisturized with an eye cream is preventative or can delay their premature deepening. Later, around the fifties, when lines are deepening around the nose and mouth and everything seems to be sagging from a lessening of elasticity, a face-lift is the only solution.

Moles
Moles are flat or slightly raised patches of dark pigmentation which can be unsightly if too bumpy or if they sprout a few hairs. The hairs shouldn't be pulled out nor should any attempt be made at home removal of the mole – they are easy to remove safely if professionally done. Most moles are harmless, but a flat mole that changes colour or size or bleeds should be medically checked immediately.

Perspiration
The body's natural heat-controlling, air-conditioning system, this is the liquid produced by the sweat-glands – regularly appearing in armpits and groin, and after exercise or specific stimulation of the

body temperature (from a sauna, for instance) occurring all over the body. The liquid is odourless but, if constricted by clothing or trapped by a fold of skin or joint, will quickly form bacteria; it is this that smells. When fresh, this smell is considered quite attractive by some, but, if allowed to become stale or dry into clothes that are worn again before being washed or cleaned, it is always unpleasant. Fat people perspire more than thin and a diet will obviously help; others come out in a 'cold sweat' from fear or emotional stress, often around the hairline and across the forehead. Excessive non-induced sweating needs medical treatment. There are excellent antiperspirants and deodorant-antiperspirants on the market, but as perspiring is a very important part of the body's natural cooling-system, you should use the mildest antiperspirant you can. Everyone differs in how much they sweat and, of course, it is a real problem for some: those who sweat excessively need the strongest possible deterrent, but most people just need a little help to control the flow and prevent a bad smell.

Red Lines
These usually appear around the nose and cheeks in the thirties and are broken surface blood-vessels caused by skin damage (windburn, frostbite), pregnancy, alcohol or high blood pressure. They can often be treated by a doctor or trained beautician inexpensively and relatively painlessly, using an electric needle and special chemical fluid to drain the blood-vessel. A serious condition, in the legs for instance, may need several sessions and take time. Later, a variety called spider angiomata, which radiate from a central red point, may appear but can be removed by cauterization.

Scars
Whenever the skin is damaged – cut, burned or stretched – it will leave a scar. Surface scars will disappear without trace (particularly in the young); deeper wounds, where the tissue is destroyed,

will leave permanent marks. Stretch marks and minor scars are sometimes helped by a vitamin E oil or special cream. Severe disfiguring ones will need chemical peeling or skin-grafting, and medical advice must be sought.

Skin Cancer

This is most commonly found in women who have spent a lifetime sunbathing without due protection for their skin. *Solar keratoses* are rough, red patches which can be surgically removed safely and will heal leaving no scar. If left untreated these pre-cancerous lesions will develop into the far more serious *squamous cell carcinoma*, which is a thickened, roughened version of the above and mostly appears on the face.

Basal cell carcinoma also appears predominantly on the face as a persistent small sore. Both these conditions can be treated by surgery or chemotherapy, but some scarring may ensue.

The most severe and fortunately rarest form of skin cancer is called *malignant melanoma* and is indicated by deeply pigmented patches, coloured brown, black or sometimes dark blue, or by a lump which suddenly changes colour when exposed to the sun. Any patch should be checked by a doctor as speedily as possible since treatment involves removal of the affected area plus a certain amount of surrounding skin, depending on the state of the growth.

Skin Discolouration

A sallow skin tone may be improved by increasing the blood circulation; likewise a pale tone. Anything that increases the flow of blood and brings more to the surface will improve the effect and give the skin a pinker tint. Regular exercises, a good brisk walk or body massage all help. A ruddy complexion is difficult to reduce – although alcohol, coffee and spicy foods should be avoided – and as far as the face is concerned, there are coloured prefoundation creams designed to help.

Sunburn

Sunburn often shows the morning after a day spent in the sun, or in the evening when the first sign is a stinging as you get into a bath. It is a painful reddening of the skin (sometimes so sensitive that even a loose cotton shirt or sheet will hurt), followed by peeling.

Very fair skins are exceptionally sensitive to the sun, but anyone – even black skins that have been away from the sun for any length of time – can on occasion suffer from sunburn and heatstroke. Very fair skins should use a sun block, wear wide-brimmed hats and cover as much of the body as possible, but everyone who values the beauty of their skin should take sunbathing gently and always wear creams that will filter out the damaging ultra-violet rays. You can still go beautifully brown: it will just take a little longer.

Unwanted Hair

Hair growing on parts of the body – face, bikini-line, underarms and legs are common – where it isn't wanted can be disguised by bleaching, which is quite satisfactory if the original growth is reasonably fair; removed temporarily with suitable depilatory creams or stripped off with wax; or removed permanently by electrolysis, which is expensive and time-consuming but worth it for a small area or if the hair is causing exceptional distress. (See also p. 57ff.)

Veruccas

Infectious inward-growing warts on the feet, usually picked up by children or young adults who frequent communal changing-rooms in schools, sports centres, swimming-pools, etc. and walk around barefoot – one verucca will soon multiply into many more – they are painful and need attention from a chiropodist, who will treat them with an acid product, electronically or, as a last resort if the verucca grows very deep, surgically.

Warts

Small hard growths appearing often on hands or face, usually on children or teenagers and mostly caused by a virus, they often just disappear, if left untreated, but if too numerous or large to leave, they can be treated with special solutions, scraped, burned or cut off. The large, soft, moist variety that occasionally appears in the genital area should be treated by a doctor.

Whiteheads

First cousin to the blackhead, they are tiny, hard, white lumps just under the skin that cannot find an exit unless the pore is opened. They should not be tampered with at home, but a trained beautician will make an opening, remove the offending waxy mass and leave not a trace.

Windburn

Red, dry patches, usually on cheeks or exposed areas, appear as a result of exposure without protection to strong winds combined with glaring light. Sportspersons, such as all-weather skiers who venture out in blizzards, dinghy and ocean-racing sailors, cross-country riders and all athletes, need to take precautions to protect their skin from windburn.

Zymotic Disease

This is a now disused and archaic description (coined by 19th-century Dr William Parr before the discovery and identification of viruses) for epidemic, endemic and contagious diseases such as smallpox that assumed the similarity of fermentation (zymosis) and infection.

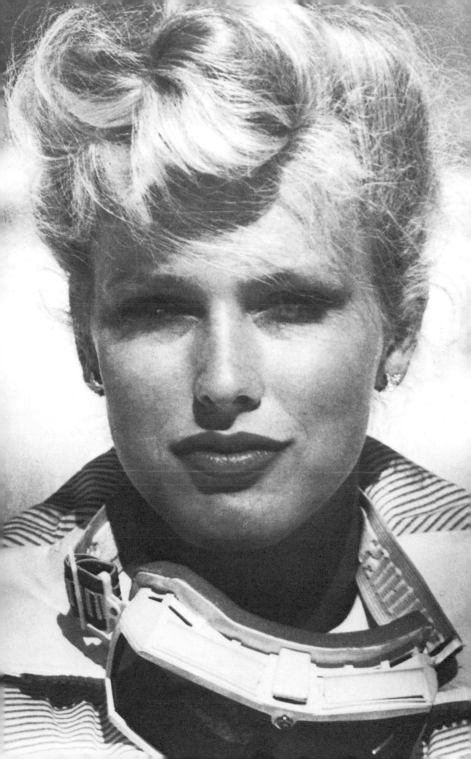

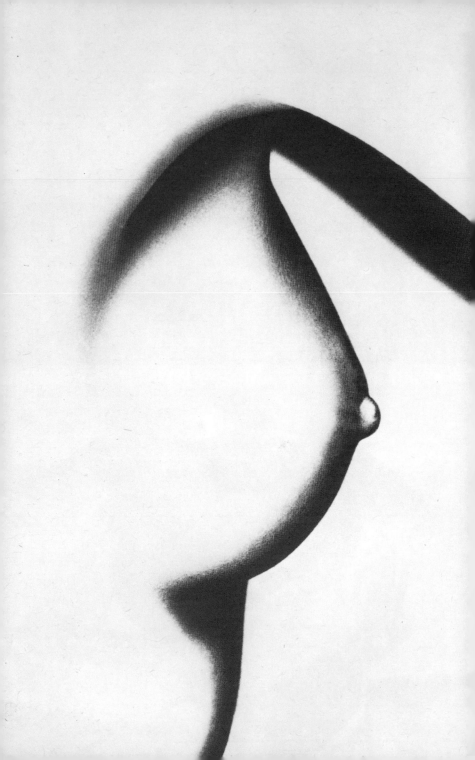

Unwanted Hair:
What to Do about It

While hair on the head is something to be admired, any profusion elsewhere on the body is in most cultures considered unattractive and something to be got rid of. Body hair is quite normal and can range from one persistent coarse hair on the chin, through a dark shadow on the upper lip, or eyebrows that meet across the bridge of the nose, to hair that grows around the nipples, under the arms, on arms, legs, fingers, toes, tummy and around the bikini-line.

There are various methods of removal to choose from.

Plucking
The easiest and most convenient way of removing stray hairs on face and breasts and it has no adverse effects, although, of course, the hair will reappear, and some people find it a slightly uncomfortable process. It is a good idea, before tweezing, to wipe the area with cotton-wool soaked in an astringent or a mild antiseptic; this will remove any oil and help you grip the smallest hair. Also, make sure you keep your tweezers scrupulously clean – wipe them also with the cotton-wool before using. Never try to remove hair that is sprouting from a mole or wart; this should be checked professionally.

Bleaching
This doesn't remove any hair but is an excellent method of disguising hair on face, arms, legs, and inner, upper thighs (the

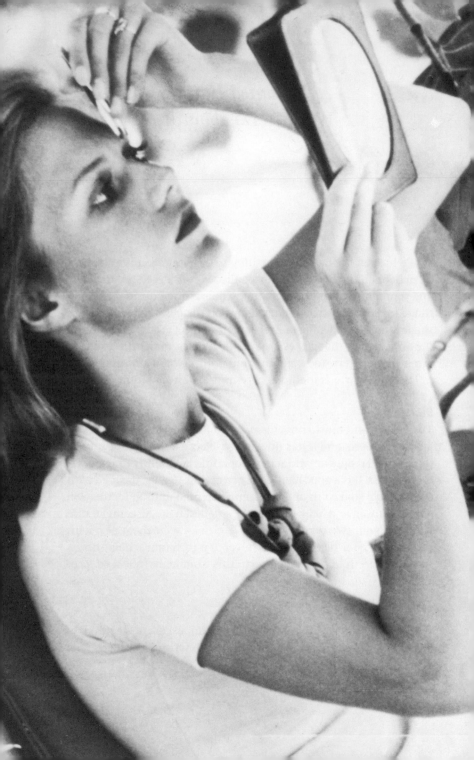

bikini area). There are good commercial products on the market, or you can make your own by mixing 30 per cent peroxide with a little ammonia and water (if you have even slightly sensitive skin, try a patch test a day in advance). Darker hair sometimes needs two applications.

Shaving

A simple and efficient way of removing underarm and leg hair, this shouldn't be used elsewhere, except where pubic hair is extending on to the upper thighs. The new hair does not grow faster or in more profusion or more coarsely, but, because it reappears with a blunt end from having been sliced off with the razor, it feels more bristly. In order to avoid cutting the skin, don't shave dry – lather the area with soap and water, use a new sharp blade and rinse and dry the skin carefully afterwards. Legs can be kept smooth with regular use of a pumice-stone – lather well, then rub the stone all over in circular movements.

Waxing

An ancient method of temporary hair removal, it is suitable for most parts of the body. (The wax is heated to a thin consistency, applied in strips, allowed to cool and then quickly ripped off, bringing the hairs with it.) It can be painful, particularly if you tend to retain water (just before getting a period, for instance), but it pulls the hair from beneath the skin's surface (although it doesn't destroy the roots) so re-growth takes longer and appears soft and smooth. Many people find that in time the re-growth is weakened and the amount of visible hair reduced. Ingrowing hairs are sometimes a problem, in which case bleaching is probably a more satisfactory method. Waxing is most efficiently done in professional salons, but wax can be bought and the process done at home; although time-consuming, it is quite satisfactory, particularly if you have a friend to help reach awkward areas.

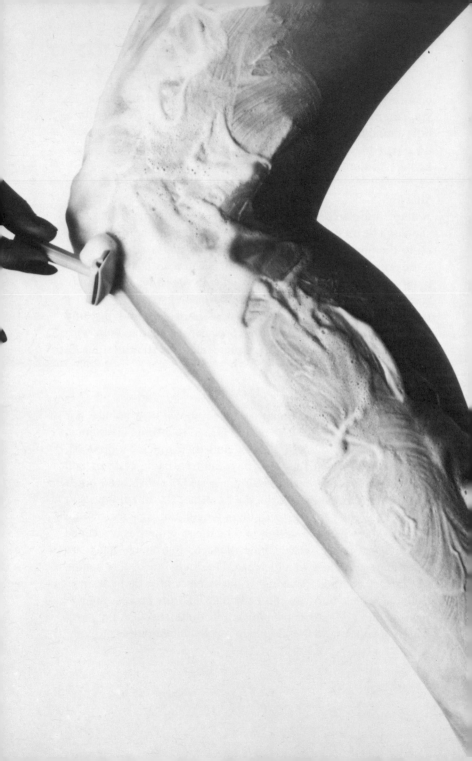

Depilation

A depilatory (a chemical normally sold as a cream, gel, powder or spray-foam) dissolves the hair shaft below the surface of the skin but doesn't destroy the root; it will sometimes weaken the hair in time, but re-growth is inevitable. There are different formulations for face and body, so make sure you buy the correct version – and, if using for the first time, try a patch test in advance and follow the directions implicitly. This method is suitable for most unwanted hair, providing the depilatory is specifically formulated for the right area.

Electrolysis

This is one of the most efficient methods and the only one offering the possibility of permanent removal, but even the best-trained technician won't guarantee there might not be some re-growth. A fine wire needle is inserted into the hair follicle and a low electric current destroys the papilla (the hair bulb) in about 40 seconds. Once the papilla is destroyed, hair from that particular bulb will never grow again. However, it is impossible to reach every papilla in an area in one session: therefore it is really only practicable for small areas (face and nipples) – legs, for instance, could take years to clear and would be extremely expensive. The pain involved varies from person to person and often depends on how close to the nerve ends the operator is working – some people just get a slight tingling sensation, others find it really hurts. But, the discomfort and expense is usually considered worth it for upper lip and chin areas and for people who are really self-conscious and distressed about an area of body hair.

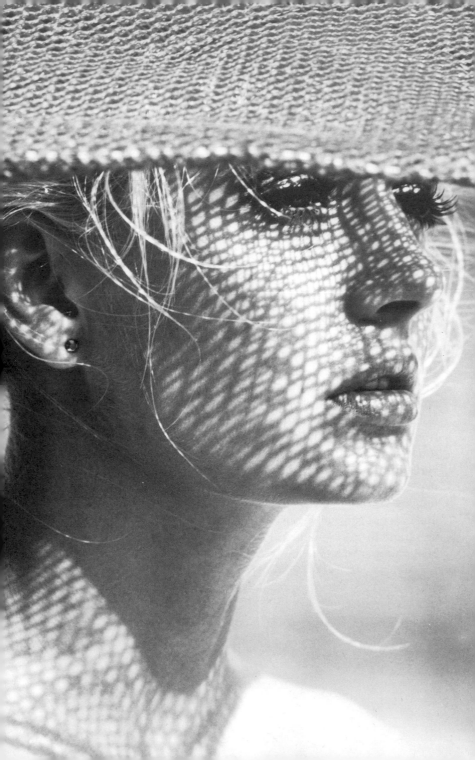

Climate:
Your Skin in the Sun and Extreme Conditions

No matter how much has been written and read about the damaging effects of the sun on skin, the world still flocks to sunny shores and slopes, and a tan is still admired ... people are thought to look 'well' with a tan; psychologically, therefore, they feel better. And it is quite possible to have a beautiful golden tan without damaging the skin, but the skin must never be allowed to *burn*, and this takes time and discipline during the first few hours and days of summer or a sunny holiday, when the excitement of blue sky and fresh air acts like adrenalin and you tend to forget all about protection and throw caution to the winds.

The fact is, the effects of too much sun on unprotected skin will sooner or later begin to show – the natural ageing process is speeded up, the skin becomes irrevocably dehydrated, looks tough and lined like leather. And, severe over-exposure can lead to heatstroke and skin cancer. So, whether you live in the sun all the time or whether you are exposed to it once or twice a year, protection is essential if you are to prolong the beauty of your skin and have the radiance that comes from a healthy tan.

Burning is caused by ultra-violet rays stimulating the pigment-bearing cells under the epidermis into producing the brown pigment called melanin. Only the shortest of these ultra-violet rays have the strength to penetrate these cells, and it will take a day or two for this action to come to the surface and produce a change of colour. This kind of tan lasts the longest. The rays with longer waves work on melanin granules already nearing the surface and turn them dark-brown. This tan lasts less time (tans don't fade, they flake off with the dead cells). The only way to prolong a tan is to slow down the natural process of shedding dead cells: moisturizing lotions and bath oils help, or the use of a self-tanning lotion (the newest ones are combined with an after-sun moisturizer). When you burn, a scorched redness will show on the skin two or three hours after exposure – because the tiny blood-vessels on the skin's surface have dilated. The next stage, depending on the severity of the burn, is for the skin to become pimply and blistered. Once the skin is burned, however lightly, peeling of the outer, damaged layer is inevitable sooner or later. Some parts of the body are particularly vulnerable – the nose and knees, for instance, because they protrude, the back of the neck and knees, because the skin there is very tender. And, if you sunbathe nude, the breasts and genitalia, of course, are the most sensitive of all.

If you want to acquire the kind of tan that is good for you and makes you glow with health, then you must have patience and protection. If you are in the sun for the first time for many months, take it slowly – avoid the midday glare completely and sunbathe for half an hour in the morning and late in the afternoon. Increase this time each day, but still avoid the hottest part and don't be misled into thinking a cool breeze off the hills or sea has taken the sting out of the sun – it is only disguising the burning rays and you still need protection. You also need protection on the water, in the water and out of the water. It's no good putting on a sunscreen first thing in the morning and believing you are safe for the day – a lot will be lost in natural perspiration, a lot more in the water and more as you dry yourself in the sun or with a towel. You must keep reapplying a sunscreen on your face and body.

Another frequent pitfall is a skiing or mountain holiday. Like sand and water, snow reflects the powerful damaging rays, and the skin can get just as burned on what seems to be a dull or hazy day as in brilliant sunshine.

Albert Watson

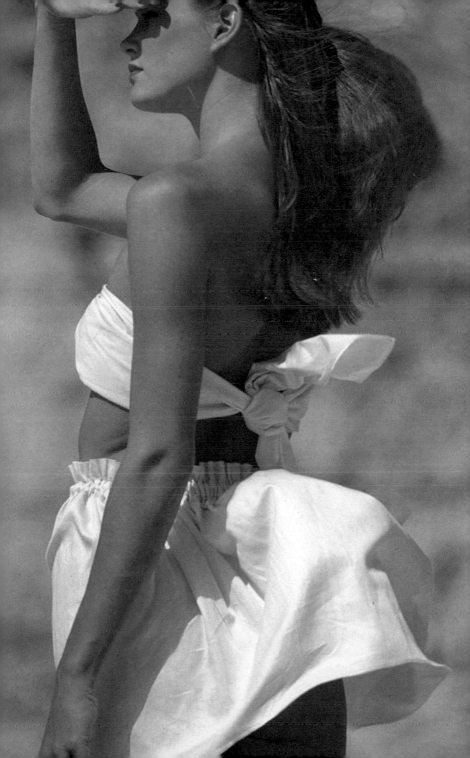

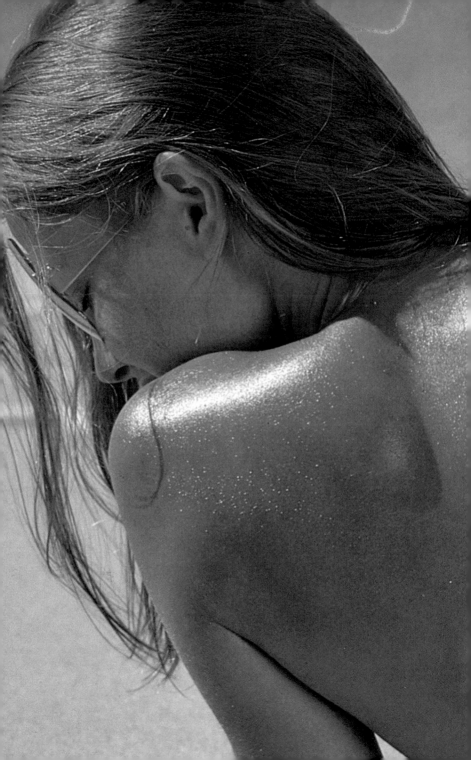

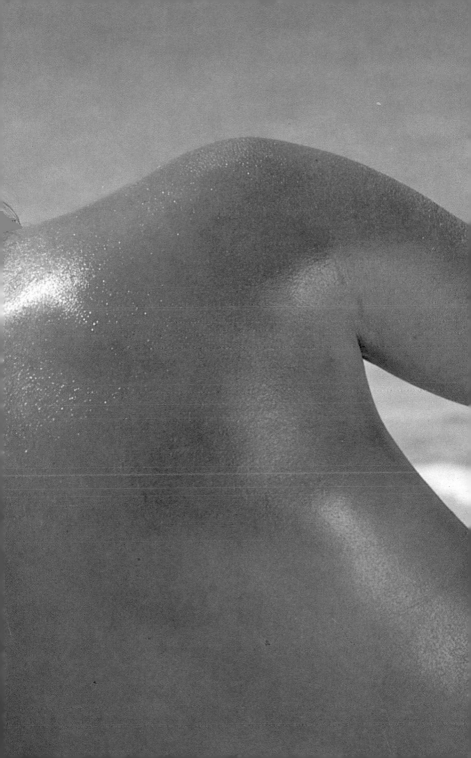

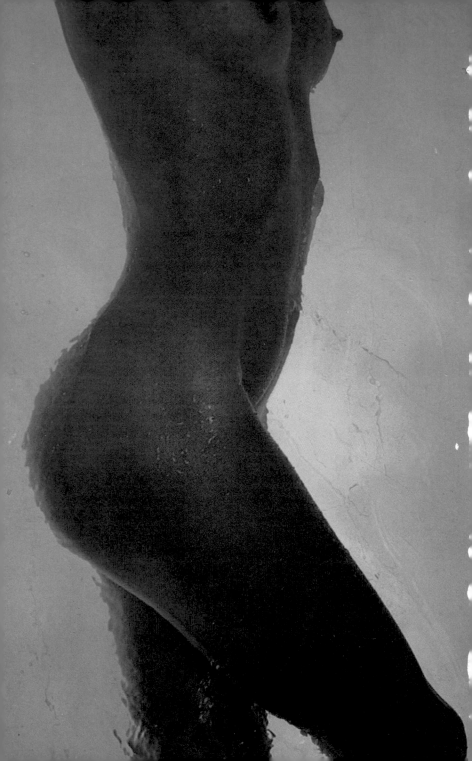

Some skins obviously burn more easily than others, but every skin needs protection to stop it from dehydrating. Very fair skin lacking in melanin will never tan deeply and red-heads with freckles just get more freckles more closely packed together. Fair skins burn quickly and take time to build a tan. Warmer-toned skins of the olive variety will be able to take more sun before burning. Brown and black skins can take even more exposure. But all skins become dryer in the sun if they are not moisturized and protected.

What to Use for Protection
Modern products range from maximum protection – sun blocks that are what they say: they block out all the rays and prevent any change of colour – to lotions, creams, gels and oils with a Sun Protective Factor (SPF) on them. To find out how long you can safely stay in the sun, you multiply the length of time it takes for your skin to burn by the SPF, e.g. if you can sunbathe five minutes before burning and you use a cream with SPF 4, you can stay in the sun safely for up to 20 minutes. If you prefer the shine of an oil to the matt absorption of a lotion or cream, be sure you choose one with a high protective ingredient; otherwise an oil is just a lubricant and provides little or no protection and will fry your precious skin. It is also wise to use a higher protective product on your face and vulnerable spots than you choose for the rest of your body. If you like to wear make-up, look for the products – foundations, lipsticks – that contain a sunscreen, and waterproof eye make-up and mascaras. The minimum looks prettiest in the sun and on a tan during the day (usually mascara and lip gloss is enough) and products with shine (frosted eyeshadows, lipsticks and blushers) look well in the evening.

Faking a Tan
The best way to have a tan and look after your skin at the same time is to use a self-tanning product that stains the skin. These are

improving all the time and, although they still need careful application so you don't get a streaky effect, this temporary staining can be very satisfactory. For best results get a friend to help you achieve an even tone and the shade you want. Some beauty salons apply a tanning treatment which lasts several days and is an excellent start to a holiday; it stops you feeling white and conspicuous and therefore being so impatient to lie in the sun that you run the risk of burning.

Sun-lamps are also good but need to be used with caution – you can burn just as badly from this artificial sunshine as from the real thing. Over a period of time, however, they prepare your skin for a sunny holiday – and will prolong that carefully acquired tan after you come home. (The latest sun *beds* claim to tan safely by filtering out the harmful rays.)

Your Skin in Extreme Climates

Travelling for most of us means more time in the sun, but extremes of cold, wind or damp need just as much consideration for the skin. In hot weather, apart from the essential sun protection discussed above, the varying types of heat may make your skin react differently.

Humidity plus air pollution. You find these conditions in large cities like New York, Rome, Tel Aviv and Tokyo. You may find your skin looks grey and dirty soon after cleansing. Your make-up fades as soon as you put it on and your skin may erupt for the first time in its life. Cities like these tend to suffer from air pollution as well as humidity in summer – and pollution constantly deposits soot and grime on the skin, demanding frequent cleansing. Use a moisturizer as a barrier between your skin and the environment; you may need to choose one for an oilier skin type than you use normally in order to keep your make-up matte and stop it from disappearing. And pack something to relieve spots, should they suddenly appear. Plus sun care, of course.

John Stember

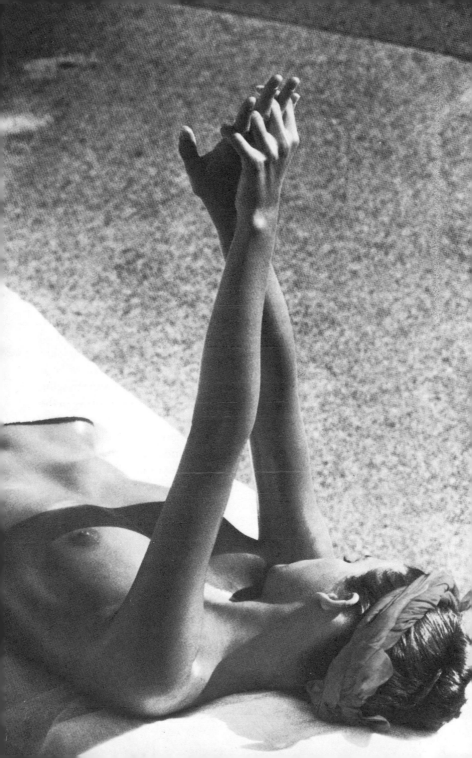

Extreme heat and aridity. Exotic spots like Marrakesh and the Nile are where you'll find this climate, and this is when skin may become extremely dry – or drier than ever before – lips parched and cracked and make-up almost impossible to apply. Take a lip emollient, a rich moisturizer for under make-up and a skin food for night-time care. Plus sun care, of course.

Tropical heat and humidity. Far-flung shores like the Seychelles, Sri Lanka and Bangkok are places to expect this climate. Skin may become excessively oily, make-up melts and hair goes limp. Keep skin extra-clean, take a good toning lotion (to refresh and tighten the texture), something to soothe spots and a moisturizer for under make-up specially formulated for oily skins (to help make-up stay put). Plus sun care, of course.

Harsh wind and extreme cold. Winter resorts such as Zermatt, Courchevel, Zurs, where high-altitude skiing is the sport, and all Polar areas are where you'll find this climate, with your skin feeling tight and dry. Use extra-rich moisturizers as well as your sun care, and avoid coming in from the intense cold and thawing out too quickly by a blazing fire – this can lead to a rupturing of the fine blood-vessels and will eventually leave red, spidery marks. Chapped skin is not a disaster and can be rehydrated with moisturizer; it usually comes from wind and is difficult to prevent if you're not going to use a thick, obvious layer of oily cream. Keep arms and legs well-lubricated too.

Albert Watson

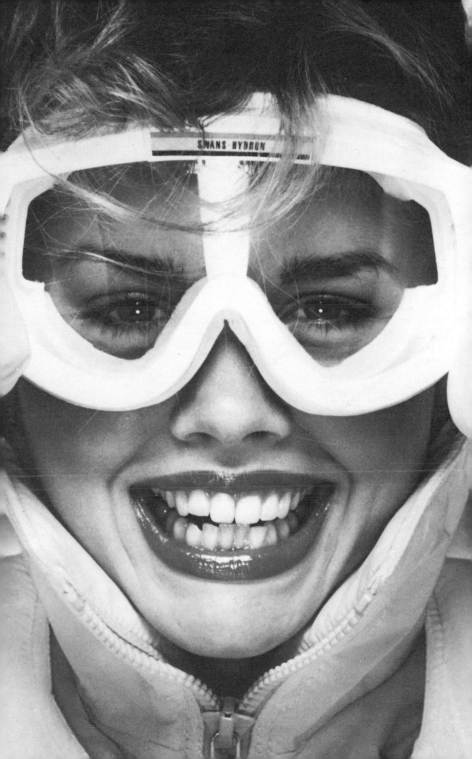

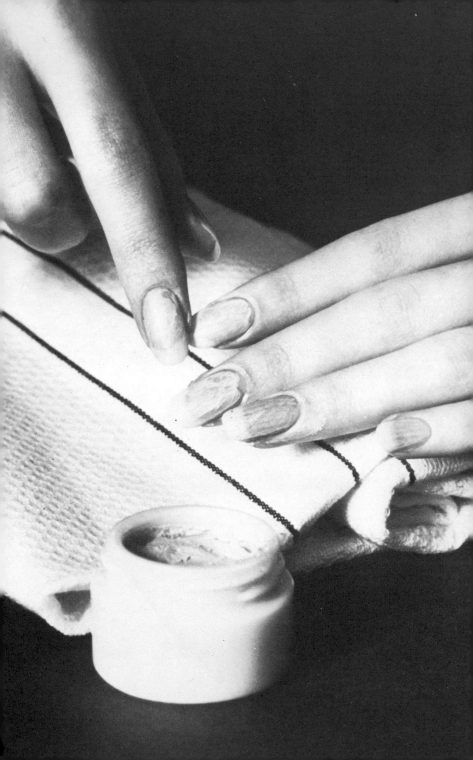

Extremities:
How to Care for Your Hands and Feet

The skin on the back of hands is fine and soft with both sebaceous and sweat-gland openings, while the skin on the palm is coarser and tougher and is one of the driest parts of the body because, unlike most other areas, it has no sebaceous glands. It does, however, have numerous sweat-glands which are often triggered off by a nervous or emotional reaction – hence the description clammy or sweaty palms – and the same is true of the soles of the feet.

Hand and wrist have great mobility from twenty-eight beautifully balanced bones. There are twenty-six bones in each foot; their strength, combined with a mass of ligaments and muscles, bears the brunt of the body weight and makes the human vertical position possible. The big toe is vital to this strength and balance as is the ball of the foot and the arch which absorbs most of the weight.

A hand can show age more quickly than any other area and, whereas surgical lifts are possible almost anywhere else, so far they have not proved successful on hands – so maintenance through care is essential. Hands that are frequently immersed in water and exposed to detergents and shampoos will dry out first. Wear rubber gloves whenever possible, always dry thoroughly and always use a hand cream afterwards. Don't neglect feet either – massage them with a good hand or body cream, paying special attention to heels and toes. Pay a regular visit to a chiropodist who will attend to patches of dry skin, corns and check for infections like athlete's foot and veruccas. This is an investment that will pay dividends by avoiding problem feet.

Manicures and pedicures are more a cosmetic treatment designed to beautify the nails, but they also keep the nail and cuticle area healthy and strong. Professional treatments are best, but you can learn to be very professional yourself and maintain finger- and toe-nails between visits. Circulation in both hands and feet is vital to their health and mobility. Here are some exercises designed to make hands more flexible and graceful, to strengthen feet and to improve circulation.

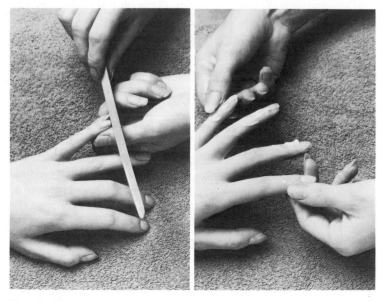

Step-by-Step Manicure

1. *File sides of the nails very gently; the ideal shape is a rounded one with straight sides. Keeping sides straight helps nails resist splitting and cracking.*

2. *Massage cuticle cream into nailbed and fingers and soak cuticles in warm water for a minute or two.*

Hand and Finger Exercises

1. Clench the fist tightly, hold a second, throw open the fingers as wide and stretched as possible. Exercise both hands simultaneously. Repeat six times.
2. Put hands straight in front of you, palms down, fingers pressed tightly against each other. Spring fingers apart as wide as possible. Repeat six times.
3. With limp, relaxed hands rotate them from the wrist in circles, first clockwise, then anti-clockwise. Turn ten circles in each direction with each hand.

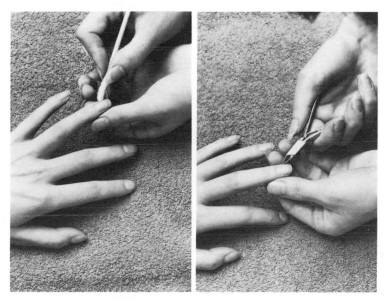

3. *Push back cuticle with orange stick wrapped in cotton wool, then with pumice stone dipped in cuticle remover (lotion).*
4. *Clip cuticle where necessary.*

4. Holding hands palms down, lift up slowly from the wrist, then lower, keeping the hands relaxed but not limp. Repeat ten times.

Useful Tips

A mask (the kind you use for your face) will cleanse, tone and moisturize your hands too.

A lemon will cleanse skin and bleach discoloured areas around nails. The lemon juice tends to dry the skin, so rinse off, dry and finish with a good massage of hand cream.

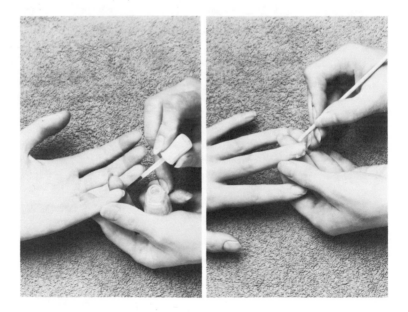

5. *Apply base coat under nail tip as well as on top of whole nail. Then wrap nail in paper nail tissue painted before wrapping with nail mender. It goes right round and under nail tip.*
6. *Prod nail tissue into place to exact shape of nail with orange stick.*

Warm olive oil is useful as a special treatment for hands, especially in winter when they are inclined to be chapped and dry. Soak them in it for about half an hour.

Cotton gloves should be worn at night whenever you can. Put them on over a layer of hand cream or petroleum jelly.

Gloves should be worn much of the time; heavy duty ones for gardening, rubber for washing activities and leather, silk or wool outside when it's cold, wet or snowing. Even in summer leather or cotton will prevent hands drying.

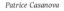

Patrice Casanova

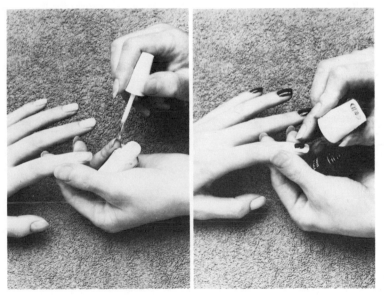

7. *Paint on another complete base coat over top of nail and tissue to seal in wrapping.*

8. *Apply an extra base coat as a top sealer which prevents polish cracking or splitting. Apply nail polish under nail tip and on top. Repeat once.*

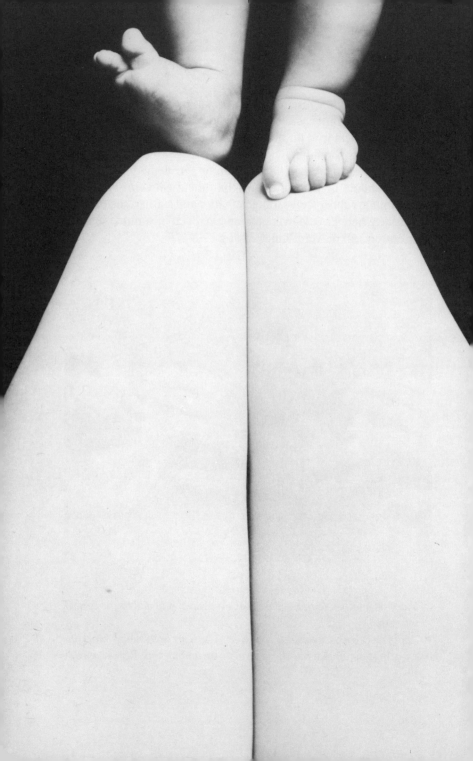

Foot Exercises

One of the best exercises of all for the feet is walking barefoot along a beach; try keeping to the water's edge, where the sand is wet. Others are:

1. Stand up straight, feet pointed ahead, and raise yourself up on your toes, then lower. This helps strengthen the foot arch and tendons around the ankle joint.

2. Cover a large book with a towel and place in front of you; with feet on book, toes extending over the edge, curl toes and try to pick up the towel. This helps strengthen the metatarsal arch, overcomes the tendency for toes to curl up and helps prevent callouses.

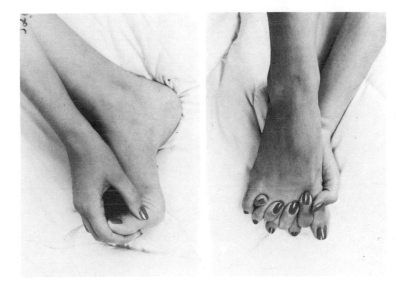

Six exercises to put you back on your feet. Spare five minutes to do them, once a day, every day.

1. Holding your foot in one hand, twist ankle inwards, then out. Repeat with the other foot. 2. Grab all your toes, bend them upwards and release. Take each toe separately and roll it around in a circle. 3. Slip

Essentials

Emery boards – for shaping nails and smoothing away hardened skin at the sides.

Pumice-stone – to soften rough cuticles or callouses and keep legs smooth.

Cuticle cream – to keep cuticles smooth and soft, avoid hangnails and encourage strong nail growth.

Orange sticks – for nudging back cuticles very gently and pushing the cuticle cream underneath.

Hand cream – to keep skin soft and supple.

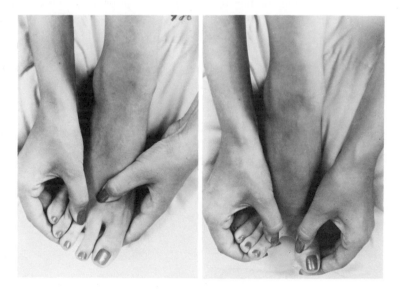

your fingers between your toes. Bend your foot down and pull it towards you. **4.** *Squeeze your foot with both hands while flexing your toes up and down. Pull each toe gently away from the one next to it.* **5.** *Press each toe firmly between thumb and index-finger, then press thumbs along the top of the foot between each of the bones at the base of the toes. Continue up to the ankle.*

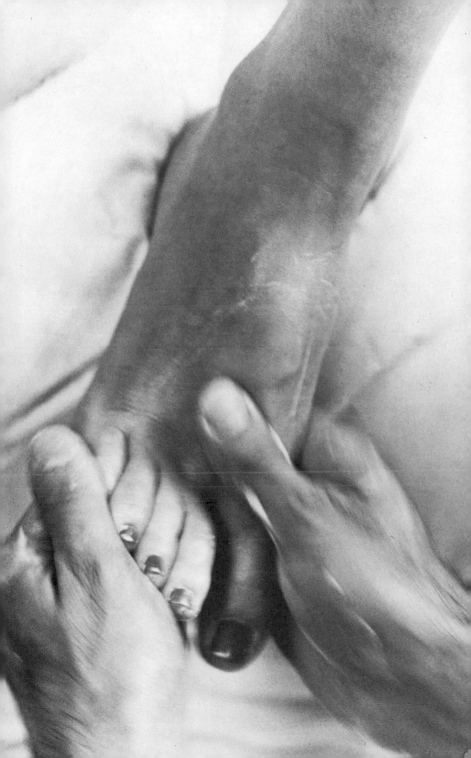

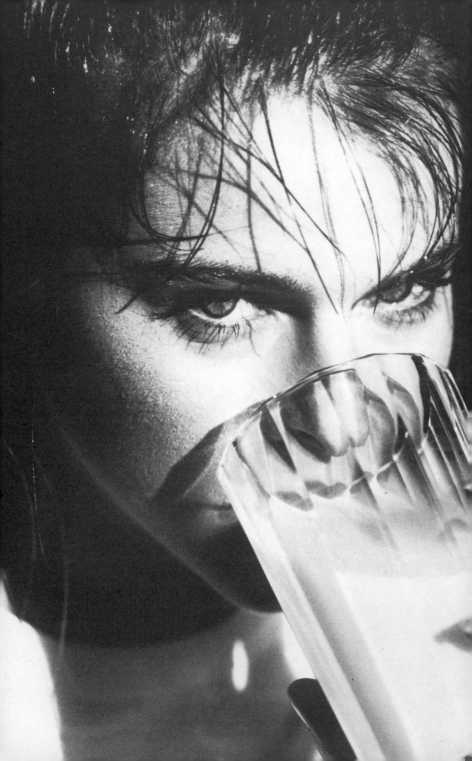

Skin Health: Eating

All skins, even healthy skins, need correct feeding and treatment, not only externally but internally. What you eat can improve or do irreparable harm to your skin. Oily skin, for example, may reflect a lack of vitamin B2 (riboflavin); this can be corrected by adding good natural food sources to your diet – liver and more milk, for instance. Oily and dimpled skin may be caused by shortage of vitamin B6 (pyridoxine). Good food sources for this include pork, veal, wheatgerm and bananas. Vitamin A is a primary skin-health vitamin and is found in dark-green and deep-yellow vegetables and fruits. Skins that are drying and ageing too soon may lack the F vitamins, pantothenic acid and niacin. Eggs and liver are excellent sources of pantothenic acid; niacin is found in beef and mushrooms.

Too much alcohol isn't good for the skin – nor is smoking. Drinking lots of water – tap or mineral – does wonders for it.

Crash diets, where the weight is removed suddenly and put back when the diet is over, are damaging to the skin and will be noticeable as you grow older, when the skin loses its elasticity and is unable to spring back. It will become flabby and lose its texture. The answer is to develop a healthy eating pattern that becomes an unbreakable habit very early in life, getting rid of any overweight gradually, so that it goes for good and the new weight is maintained. Try to avoid fatty foods, highly spiced foods, sweets, cakes, biscuits, sauces and too many rich dairy foods; learn to like fresh fruit, salads and vegetables, grilled fish and meat and wholewheat bread. A diet high in these items and water, and low in the others and alcohol, will keep your skin in good shape for a lifetime.

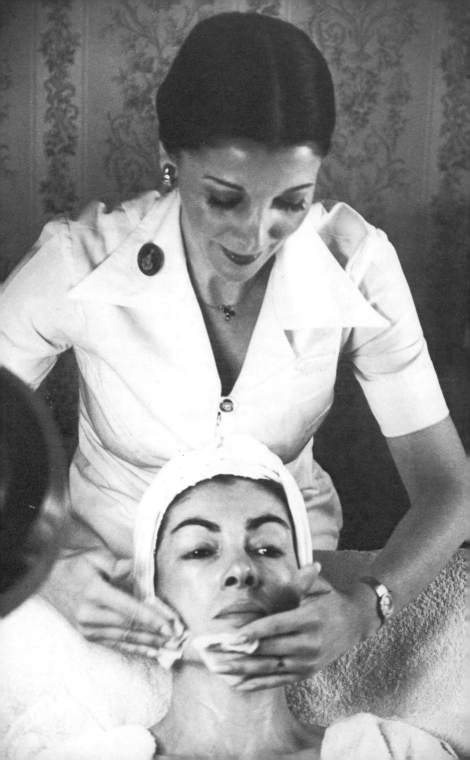

Professional Skin Treatments:
Face and Body

Professional treatments range from a cleansing facial in a beauty salon through massage and skin peeling to cosmetic plastic surgery. Considered by some as an extravagant indulgence, they can do much to help beauty both on a mostly psychological short-term basis, and in the long term, by an extension of the youthful qualities of the skin and body.

Face
Professional facials. Theories differ about the benefits of massaging the face, and it is a matter of personal opinion, but a deep-cleansing treatment can do nothing but good. Personal recommendation is a good way of finding an expert beautician, and it is important that you like the feel of their hands and get on well with them because the relaxation that should be part of the treatment is vital to the results. It is also important that the products smell and feel pleasant to you – who wants to close their eyes for twenty minutes under, what is to them, an evil-smelling mask? After a cleansing treatment it is usually recommended that no make-up is worn for a day – or twenty-four hours if possible – to give the skin a chance to breathe and make the most of its new vitality. So, make an appointment with that in mind. Facials also help to reduce wrinkles.

Wrinkles – or lines – are one of the first signs that skin is beginning to age and usually appear around the eyes or mouth, caused by premature dehydration in these delicate areas. There are new creams coming on the market all the time as a result of constant research into this problem and, although none will eliminate the lines, many of them help prevent their deepening and multiplying too fast. Professional facials often help too, with the use of special oils, emollients, massage and masks. But the only way to soften or remove them is through *peeling* – or dermabrasion. These are medical procedures carried out by doctors or highly qualified beauticians. They are an extension of cosmetic exfoliating – the removal of dead surface cells from the skin by means of an abrasive cream, gel or lotion applied with a brush or rough-textured pad. The result is better-textured skin with a more even tone. As skin grows older and lines begin to deepen, the only way to help is by literally removing the top layer of skin and revealing the new one underneath. This is done either by chemical surgery or by dermabrasion, the latter method of *planing* often being used on scars, as it can be done on small areas. Both methods take from three to six months before the final improvement is visible.

Plastic surgery is the most drastic method of improving or prolonging the youthful aspects of face and body, the cosmetic possibilities being realized after the science was pioneered during the war in rebuilding badly burned and scarred servicemen. Only carried out by highly qualified surgeons, these operations can restructure for life features like noses, ears or chins; reduce fatty areas by removing the fatty deposits from under the surface or taking part of the skin and bone away; or improving shape by adding bone or silicone. Wrinkles, lines and sagging skin are smoothed and tightened by lifting and tucking away. Successful operations are now carried out on: breasts, buttocks, chins, ears, eyes, face, neck, nose, stomach and thighs.

How long they last depends on the individual – age, inherited problems, stress and how much care is taken with diet, exercise, skin and sun care after treatment.

Body

Plastic surgery is a drastic and often expensive means of improving body shape and texture, but operations like breast enlargement are usually very rewarding. A good exercise routine, started early in life and practised regularly, can do much to improve posture and shape and keeps muscles working, so that the body is supple and graceful.

Massage is enormously beneficial to the body – the gentle, kneading strokes revitalizing muscles, decreasing tension and stimulating circulation. It is a great tranquillizer – some people actually fall asleep during the massage – and, as most masseurs use an emollient cream or oil, the skin benefits too. In conjunction with a slimming diet and exercise, massage will help get rid of overweight and reshape the body. As with beauticians, it is important to find a masseur that suits you – although the methods may be basically the same, individuals develop their own special routines, using more or less pressure, for instance, and choosing special oils for their aroma or therapeutic values.

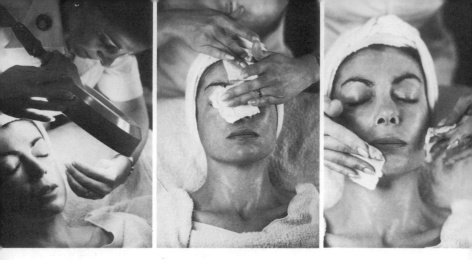

Step-by-Step Deep Cleanse Treatment

This is a professional cleansing treatment that nourishes and re-balances the skin, improving elasticity and tone, softening wrinkles. Originally conceived to help acne, it was discovered that this method, using a galvanic/high-frequency machine, was equally good for general skin care. The treatment is here undergone by the author.

1. The skin is examined to establish its type and which products to use. 2. The skin is cleansed with a suitable product: here, one for sensitive skin with broken veins. 3. The skin is toned with a suitable product and the face is blotted dry with tissue. 4. The skin is re-examined and blackheads and sebum removed. 5. A special solution,

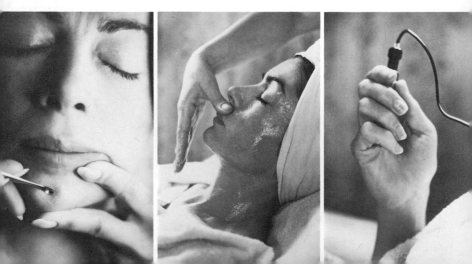

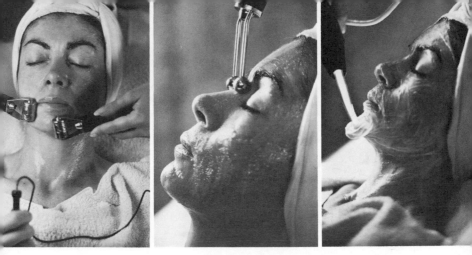

Electro Z, is used to help overcome the skin's natural resistance to electric current and catiogenic gel is smoothed over face and neck. **6.** *A small metal bar is held; this makes the skin receptive to the galvanic current. The machine is switched on and the current adjusted.* **7-9.** *Roller applicator heads are passed over the skin's surface to loosen accumulated grease and dirt in the pores; a light perspiration is set up, which rejects the dirt.* **10.** *The machine is switched to high frequency and oxygen cream and gauze are spread over to boost the effect of the treatment.* **11.** *The face is massaged with a liquid to contract the pores, nourish and regenerate the skin. A mask is then chosen, suitable for the type of skin.* **12.** *The mask is cleaned off, the skin toned and moisturized. The fresh clean skin should not be made-up for twenty-four hours.*

Sandra Lousada

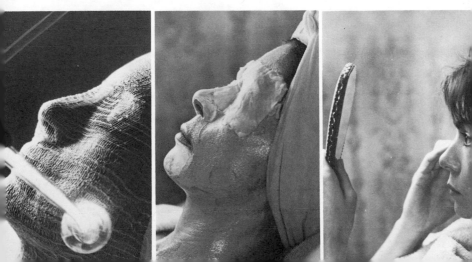

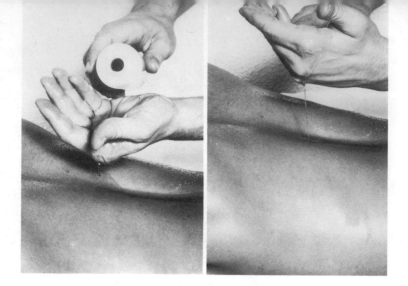

There is still nothing more effective after a hot sauna than a professional massage to revive one. One of the oldest methods, although little practised in Europe, is the Shiatsu – an extremely relaxing technique of applying pressure to one's nerve endings, which automatically releases all muscular pain, stress and tension.

An added bonus with massage, by traditional or modern methods, is the dislodging of fat cells. By stimulating circulation it disperses fatty deposits and rejuvenates the skin.

The photographs show the masseur concentrating on the area of the back that causes most trouble.

Renato Grignaschi

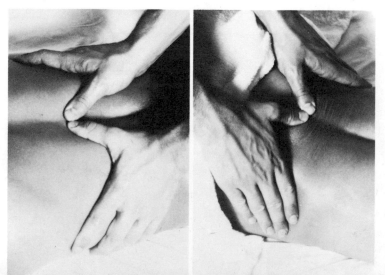

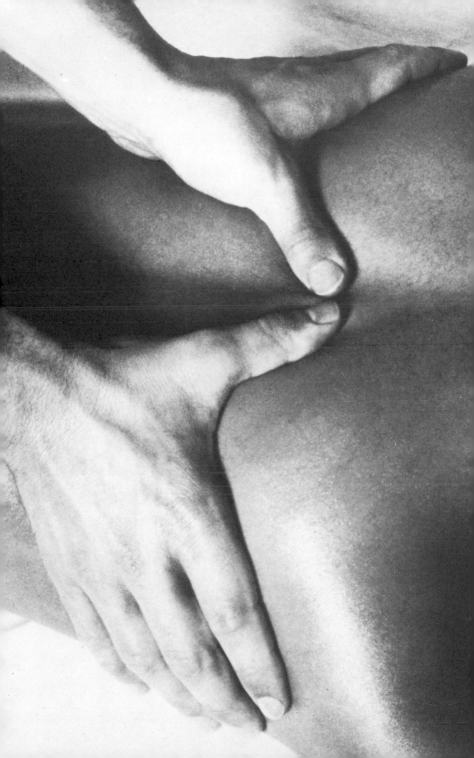

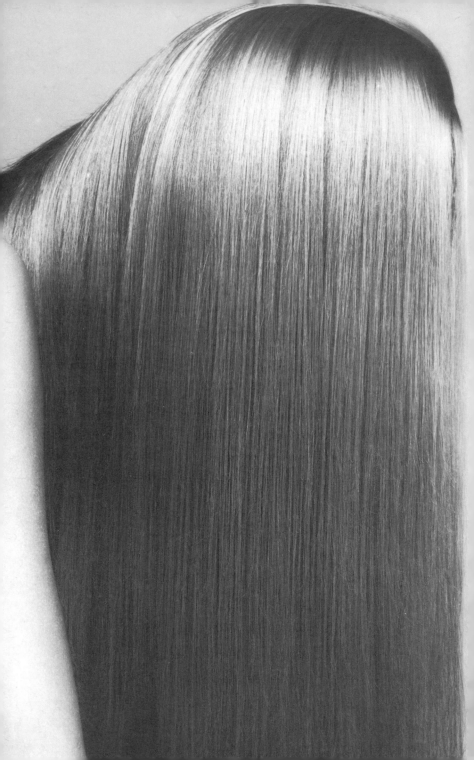

What is Hair?

Most people have around 100,000 strands of hair on their head – some may have a few thousand less, some many thousands more, but this is the average, whatever the texture. Red-heads, although they have the thickest hair, have the least strands; brunettes come next; and blondes, with the finest hair, have the most strands. Paradoxically, blond hair can often look limp and thin while red hair looks abundantly thick. Each strand starts below the surface of the skin in a little nodule known as the *papilla*, which, even when a hair is plucked out 'by the roots', is left behind to start again and eventually produce a new hair. The *root* is the section of the hair below the skin's or scalp's surface – the visible part above, whatever its length, is the *shaft*. The root is enclosed in a sac called the *hair follicle*, the base of which forms the papilla. Each strand, even though the outward appearance may vary from person to person, has the same basic structure of three layers. The innermost layer or *medulla* is soft and spongy, providing a small amount of colour from cells sometimes containing granules of colour pigment; this is surrounded by the *cortex*, composed of long thin cells, which provides elasticity and most of the colour; lastly there is the outer layer, or *cuticle*, which consists of overlapping scales designed to protect the other two layers. The papilla receives a blood supply enabling it to produce the hair. The quality of this blood determines the strength of the hair. It makes sense, therefore, to make sure that your daily diet includes not only the vitamins and minerals essential for a healthy body, but those particularly beneficial to hair, i.e., lots of protein (hair is 97% protein, 3% moisture) and vitamin B (Brewers' Yeast tablets are a good source of this) – and to cut down on sugar, salt and animal fats. The diet that is good for healthy hair is good for the rest of you.

The minute the hair leaves the follicle, i.e., when it shows on the surface and becomes the shaft, it is, to all intents and purposes, dead. It is no longer receiving nourishment from the papilla and its health and condition will depend on outside help. This period of 'rest' in the life-span of the hair strand will continue for as much as six years, until it eventually falls out and is replaced by a new hair manufactured in the same papilla. The growth cycle is 'staggered' from hair to hair and distributed over the scalp, so that when hairs fall out through this natural process it is unnoticeable in the general amount of hair on the head; up to a hundred hairs a day should be accepted as quite normal. Only when daily 'fall-out' is abnormally large should it be seen as a warning signal and steps be taken to locate the cause and treat it.

There are oil-glands attached to the hair follicles secreting natural oils, but not enough to reach far along the shaft; once the hair grows to any length, the ends certainly never get fed. This

RIGHT: *A highly magnified photograph illustrating the thread-like fibres within the inner structure or the cortex of the hair.*

OPPOSITE LEFT: *A highly magnified shot of a hair that has been damaged by improper care. It illustrates how the layers of the cuticle have separated and shows how easily this hair would become entangled during styling and thus be harder to work on than healthy undamaged hair.*

OPPOSITE RIGHT: *A microscopic enlargement of a split hair. There is no known chemical remedy to heal a 'split end' and it can only be cured by cutting it off.*

Wella International

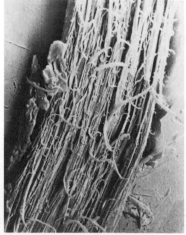

means, of course, that the ends become starved as they get older and are most vulnerable to damage. Cutting off dry brittle ends will stop them from splitting and leave the hair looking fuller and healthier – and sometimes give the impression of faster-growing hair. This, however, is an illusion – it is not possible to alter the hair's growth-pattern, which is fixed when you are conceived. The average growth is around half an inch (1·3 cm) a month, which slows as you grow older, and, although individuals may have a faster or slower growth-rate, it is not affected by cutting the hair. Some people have difficulty growing their hair to any length at all while others seem to get it to reach their waist in no time. This is because of the combination of growth-rate and life-span: hair that seems hardly to grow at all combines a slow growth-rate with a short life-span; those lucky enough to possess a fast growth-rate with a long life-span can grow long hair quickly. This combination, like the texture of your hair, is hereditary and there is nothing you can do to alter it. The colour and curliness of your hair, although also determined by ancestry, can be changed with modern chemicals.

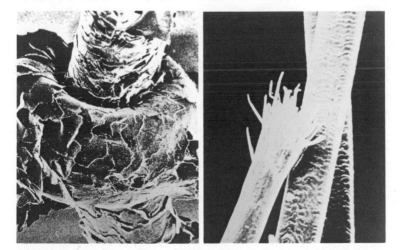

Hair Types

If your hair doesn't please you, it will affect the way you look and feel. So the more you know about your type of hair, the more you'll be able to do with it and the less you'll try to expect impossible things from it. The first and most important thing you need to know is what type of hair you have. Is it oily, dry or mixed? Has it been permed or straightened? Has the colour been altered by tinting or bleaching? You need to answer all these questions before working out a hair-care routine. Next, you need to study its thickness and texture and curling ability to determine the variety of styles in which it will behave well and, bearing in mind the shape of your face, height, weight and life-style, eliminate those that are unsuitable. The combination of correct hair-care routine plus suitable hair style will make sure you are getting the maximum from this vital part of your beauty image.

Oily Hair
Oily hair almost always goes with oily skin and frequently with fine hair. A certain amount of oil is vital for hair and skin, but when the oil-glands produce more than can be absorbed problems begin. Oily hair is easily recognizable as it becomes lank soon after shampooing and then quickly looks greasy and in need of another wash.

It used to be thought that frequent shampooing stimulated the glands into producing even more oil, but current thinking is that a clean scalp is essential to the control of greasy hair and, providing the correct shampoo is used, it doesn't matter even if it is washed as much as twice a day. The rule is: wash whenever your hair looks or feels in need.

For oily hair, use the mildest, blandest shampoo you can find. Use the shampoo sparingly, wash your hair and scalp gently – don't scrub or over-massage – and rinse scrupulously, finishing with cold water. Sometimes greasy hair needs conditioning, but only if the ends are dry or split – in this case, apply conditioner only on the dry ends and use as little as possible, rinsing off well. After shampooing or between shampoos it helps to cleanse the scalp with an astringent lotion. The method is to part the hair in sections, soak a cotton-wool ball in the lotion and wipe it down the partings – until you have covered the whole scalp; witch-hazel and the juice of a lemon diluted in water are excellent. Diet is important in the control of greasy hair – cut out animal fats, fried foods, carbohydrates, eggs, nuts, alcohol, salad dressing. Step up intake of low-fat protein (like white fish or chicken), raw vegetables, salads and fresh fruit and drink lots and lots of water.

Dry Hair
Dry hair occurs when too little oil is secreted from the glands attached to the hair follicle or the hair shaft is damaged by bleaching or frequent exposure to the elements – wind, sun, salt or chlorine-filled water or central heating, all of which cause the natural moisture to evaporate. If dry hair is a permanent problem, the sufferer will probably have dry skin too, but if it is caused by external damage to the hair shaft, particularly by bleaching, it could be combined with any skin type (although over-exposure to harsh elements causes devastating damage to skin too). Dry hair is hard to control, full of electricity and lacks lustre, with little ends sticking up all over the place. Permanent or hereditary dry hair is not helped by infrequent shampooing. You might think that shampooing washes away the natural oils and dries out the hair even further, but in fact lack of washing only results in a dirty

scalp. Dry hair, like all hair conditions, needs a clean scalp to allow the hair follicles and sebaceous glands to function with maximum efficiency – and shampooing and conditioning with the correct products is essential. Self-inflicted dry hair – caused by over-bleaching, over-tinting or over-exposure to outside elements – is easier to treat because the problem is with the hair shaft, which is continually being renewed, and not with the papilla, where the hair is formed. Dandruff, in severe cases, can cause dry hair. This is often because, in an attempt to cure the dandruff, the wrong shampoo is being used, which prevents the natural oils from reaching the base of the hair shaft. You should find a shampoo specially formulated for dry hair and always use a conditioner. An oil treatment once or twice a week before shampooing can do wonders too: warm some olive oil or a light vegetable oil and part the hair down the middle; apply from forehead to nape, then work down the sides in sections until the whole head is saturated. Use your fingers to massage the oil into the scalp and hair, then wrap your hair in plastic (cling-film is excellent) and cover with a towel, preferably warm, which will cause moisture to build up under the plastic. The longer you can leave this treatment on, the better; overnight is ideal. In the morning the oil can be removed by two washes with shampoo. A correct diet is essential in treating permanent and self-inflicted dry hair – you need to ensure that the blood feeding the papilla is rich enough and that there is enough oil in your system, so step up your intake of low-cholesterol polyunsaturated oils (eat margarine, make salad dressings from sunflower oil or light vegetable oils, eat low-fat cheese and yogurt), raw vegetables and fruit, take a supplement of vitamin E oil capsules and cut down on carbohydrates, alcohol and spicy foods.

Mixed Condition Hair

Mixed condition hair is the combination of an oily scalp with dry hair. The scalp may *feel* dry and be flaking with dandruff scales, but the hair shaft is drying out because the oil secreted from the glands

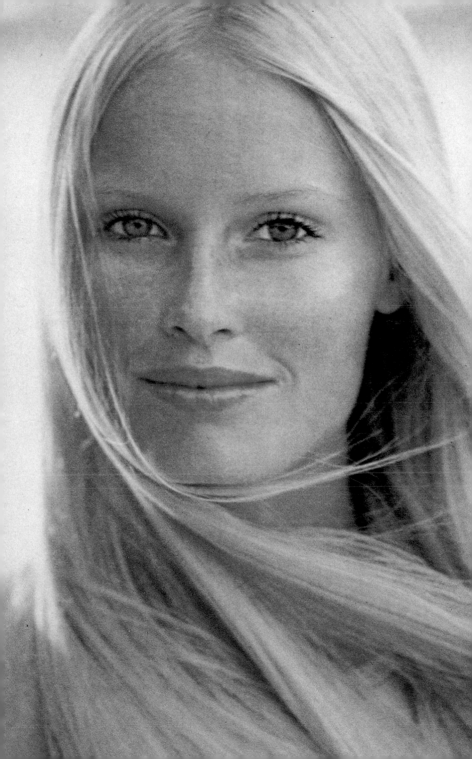

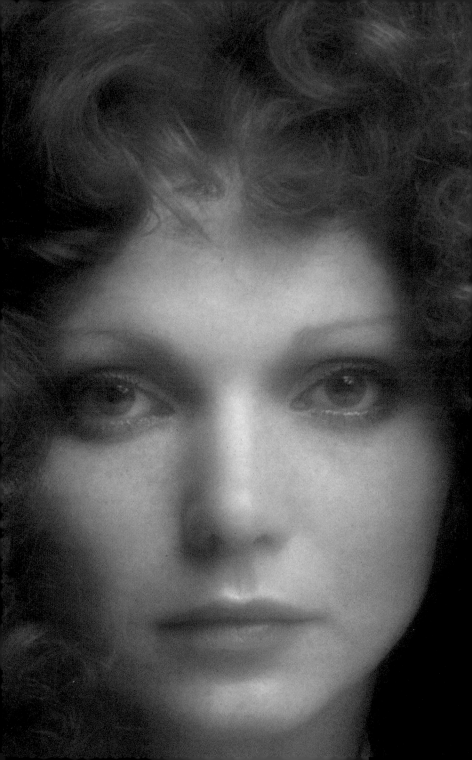

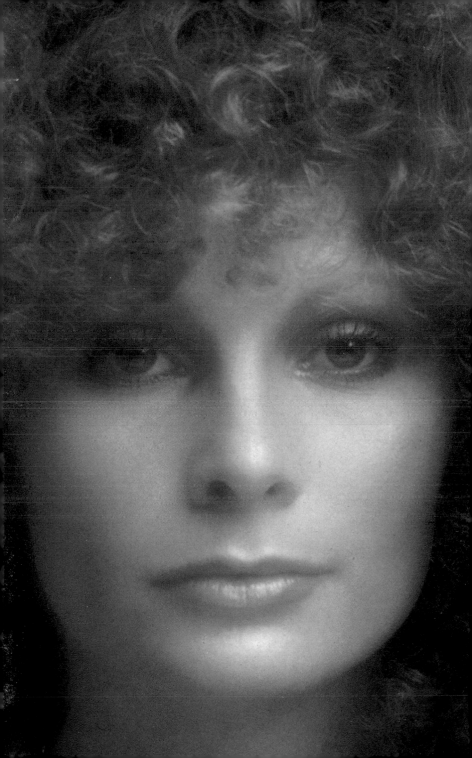

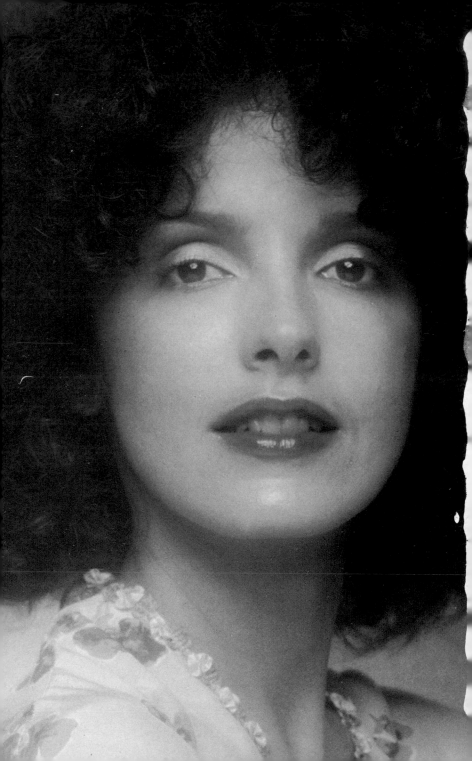

in the follicle is soaking into the dandruff flakes, clogging the follicle and preventing the flow of oil along the hair shaft.

The first step to cure this condition is to clear the scalp of flaking scales by using a mild anti-dandruff shampoo or a lotion applied after the head has been shampooed and conditioned. After the scaling has cleared, use a shampoo for dry hair, a conditioner and then an astringent or anti-dandruff lotion to ensure that the scalp remains clear. Avoid animal fats, fried foods, carbohydrates, eggs, nuts, alcohol, salad dressings – and concentrate on low-fat protein (white fish, chicken), raw vegetables, salads, fresh fruit (no bananas) and lots of water.

Balanced or Normal Hair

This is the ideal hair condition, one that everyone strives and longs for. Balanced hair is shiny, well-behaved and doesn't cry out for washing too frequently. The scalp is clear, the sebaceous glands producing the right amount of oil to flow along the shaft, and probably the rest of the body is in excellent order too – a balanced, nutritious diet is followed, regular exercise is taken and the facial skin is in good condition. However, even this hair will not remain wonderful for long if it is not given due care and attention. A careless holiday in the sun, a course of antibiotics (or other medication), a binge of overeating, a broken limb causing in-activity, a bad perm or tint – any of these can upset the delicate balance of the scalp and hair and cause problems.

Use a mild shampoo as often as necessary; always condition and rinse thoroughly; after the hair has been exposed to any stress (sun or wind, for instance), give it a deep conditioning treatment.

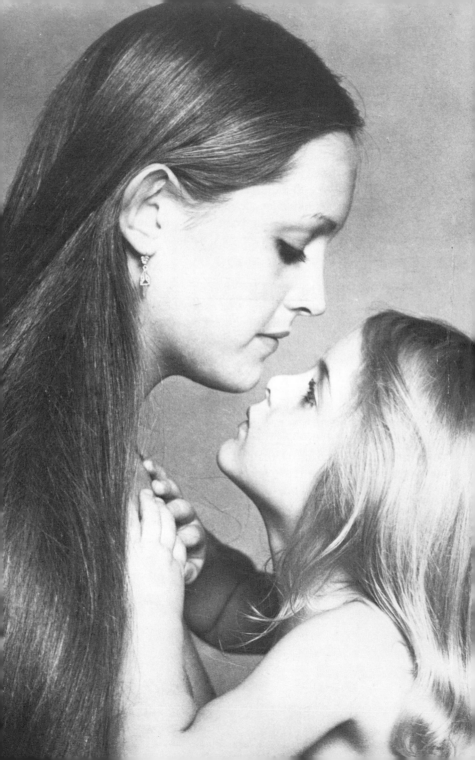

What Happens to Hair at What Age?

From Birth to Ten

The amount of hair on your head is decided before you are born, and the size of the circumference of each follicle is fixed irrevocably. The pregnant woman cannot alter the amount of hair her child will be born with or its type or texture, but she can, by taking proper care of herself and eating nutritious food, ensure that her child's hair has the best possible start.

Fewer follicles than the average doesn't necessarily mean that the hair will be thinner, because the diameter of each follicle may be wider in compensation, causing the hair shaft to be thicker. People with thin hair usually have the most hair follicles, those with thick hair the least. Babies are often born with a considerable amount of hair which falls out in the first few weeks and then begins to grow again.

The age at which a baby starts growing hair varies from child to child, but by the time it is three or four you will know what type of hair it will have. Every time a small baby is bathed its scalp should also be washed and this routine can be a very healthy one to carry on throughout life; mothers should be taught to avoid putting any pressure on the soft spot at the crown (the fontanelle) that babies are born with but not to be so frightened that they don't wash it at all! Lack of routine washing of the scalp can cause a condition known as *cradle cap* – this is a brownish, scaly patch which can spread all over the baby's scalp if not checked by treatment. It can also be caused by a fault in feeding. Cradle cap is treated with warm oil (olive, nut or light vegetable); soak cotton wool in the oil and dab it lightly over the scalp, then wash off with baby soap.

When the child's hair is grown and its type determined, choose a suitable shampoo and conditioner, wash frequently and keep an eye on the scalp and hair for any changes in condition due to climate, environment or age.

Problems: children's heads, even in this day and age, can become infested with fleas and lice – more prevalent in long hair than short; if this happens, go to a doctor for treatment. Ringworm is another infection that children are susceptible to up to the age of puberty. It looks like a circular scaly patch, about half an inch in diameter, sometimes with a pinkish centre; again the child should be taken to the doctor for treatment.

The better balanced a child's diet, the better chance it has of healthy hair – junk food, sugar and too many dairy products are all as detrimental to hair as they are to general body health. If a child can be persuaded to *like* fruit, fruit juices, raw or dried fruits and yogurt instead of sugar-based drinks, sweets, crisps and ice-creams, it will feel enormous benefit for the rest of its life.

The Teens
The hormonal changes that occur with puberty can have a dramatic effect on hair. The male and female hormones pouring through a child's bloodstream cause hair to appear on parts of the body other than the head. Boys need to start shaving, girls start thinking about unwanted hair on legs, underarms and lips. Both sexes develop pubic hair.

It is a time of tremendous activity in the body and at the same time the adolescent is often under pressure and studying for important exams. Stress can be reflected in the health of hair at any time, but it is most likely in the teens.

Hormonal changes often cause oily hair, the glands being stimulated into over-production of oil, which floods the hair shaft, gives an overall effect of lank greasiness and often produces a bad odour. The hair should be washed every day – twice a day, if necessary – with a shampoo formulated for oily hair; if a conditioner is used, only apply it to the ends. To prevent odour, all oily and fatty foods, sugar, salt, spice and dairy products must be avoided; if he or she is a junk-food addict, this habit must be broken. Dandruff is another problem often first encountered at this time and care must be taken that the dandruff treatment does not aggravate the oily condition of the hair. The cause of this dandruff is often tension and (as with oily hair) the treatment is to alter diet and encourage scrupulous cleansing of the scalp. Extra vitamin B will often help. In mild cases a shampoo for oily hair will usually control the dandruff, but severe cases may need special treatment such as a medicated shampoo containing sulphur or zinc pyrithione.

Problems: split ends are very prevalent amongst teenagers – often caused by over-enthusiastic use of electrical equipment. In finding hair styles that suit and in keeping pace with changing moods, teenagers overuse blow driers, heated rollers, styling brushes and curling tongs. They are impatient and feel they haven't the time to let their hair dry gently with the dryer on 'low' – everything is done at top speed and on the highest setting, which is fine for saving time but disaster for the hair: a too-hot dryer can burn the scalp and dry out the hair shaft; heated rollers taken out in a hurry can tangle the hair really badly and, if used too often, dry out the ends. The answer for split ends is to cut them off – if you catch them soon enough it makes little difference to the overall length of hair – and never allow them to spread right up the hair shaft. It is better still to prevent them appearing by using electrical aids carefully and making sure the hair is well conditioned and not allowed to dry out. *Trichotillomania* is the term for the mania for pulling out one's own hair to the extent of causing bald patches – girls of eleven to fourteen and menopausal women are susceptible. It is thought to have two main causes: an unconscious need for masochistic sexual gratification, a side-effect of sexual fantasies; or an unconscious need for extra attention from someone close. The cure is to find the cause – in the first case, the child will probably soon grow out of the habit; in the second, extra understanding of the teenager's confused state of mind, tolerance of unpredictable moods and patient kindness will probably do the trick, but in either case a visit to a qualified trichologist will help.

The Twenties

The twenties should be a time of maximum health in every respect. Hormones have settled down, adolescent problems are over, the body should be in peak condition, worries about ageing a long way off and all the excitement of the future ahead. But, on the negative side, this is when many women start to abuse their hair by over-colouring, perming, straightening – *anything* to be fashionable! – and when sun and wind damage begin to be noticeable after a few years of regular holidays in the sun, on the sea or skiing. Many women become pregnant in their twenties and may suffer from hair loss either during pregnancy or shortly after the birth – or this may happen with a second or third child for the first time. The prime concern of the body is to nourish the unborn child and, if the woman's diet is low in essential nutrients, like iron, calcium, and protein, there may be insufficient blood, oxygen and food nutrient supplies to satisfy the unborn child, its mother and her hair. Pregnancy hair loss cannot be prevented, but proper care and diet will reduce the quantity and ensure healthy regrowth.

Sun damage – either from summer or winter sun – demands instant re-conditioning. A good treatment is warm olive oil (or a light vegetable oil) applied to the hair, massaged in and covered in plastic film. Wrap the head in a warm towel and leave for as long as possible – overnight is ideal – before shampooing out. Then try to prevent the damage recurring by taking preventative steps: cover your hair with a scarf in wet or windy weather; rinse out salt- or chlorine-filled water immediately, then shampoo and condition; use protective lotions on your hair before going out in the sun.

Oily hair occurring at this age is normally due to a bad washing routine, incorrect shampoo or a persistently poor diet. Don't wash in hot water, but use warm: rinse in cooler water, finishing with a cold rinse; try a less rich shampoo and make sure it is designed for oily hair; check diet for a high intake of fatty, sugary or spicy foods and cut them out.

Coarse hair can be a problem in the twenties, when the extra oils produced in adolescence have subsided, leaving the coarse hair in a drier, bushier condition. Wash with a shampoo for dry hair, condition with a cream rinse, combing it with a wide-toothed comb, and comb the hair into place while it's still wet and pliable.

The Thirties

Hair may start to dry out as the oil-producing glands begin to slow down; regular, richer hair-conditioning treatments will improve its health. Dryness may also be the result of years of bleaching, colouring and permanent waving; after many of these processes it is essential to re-condition the hair, as the harsh chemicals will have stripped it of most of its natural oil and moisture, leaving the hair shafts lack-lustre and brittle.

Hair loss is often a by-product of stress in the thirties. Career or marriage problems, responsibilities of parenthood, all begin to pile up; one of the first signs of this sort of tension is hair loss. If the stress is reduced, hair will regrow, because the papilla is only waiting for the right conditions to start manufacturing again. But if the stress continues and becomes worse the hair loss will become more serious and treatment for both conditions is essential. Poor health can also cause hair loss, for while the body is using all its resources to recover from illness it cannot nourish the hair.

Grey hairs can appear at any age, but by thirty most people have a few and are wondering why. Each strand of hair contains *melanin*, or colour granules, and those which have no melanin at all are white. Some people are born with white strands, some teenagers acquire them at puberty, but mostly they begin to appear as the hair ages. As with all other forms of ageing, certain processes slow down, and in this case it is the formation of colour pigment in the cortex of the hair shaft. As the colour pigment fails to form, it is replaced with air space, making the hair strand appear white or grey. The grey effect comes from the mixture of white and coloured hairs. Heredity plays a part in deciding when you will start going grey; it is thought that stress and worry and lack of vitamins such as vitamin B, which is essential to healthy hair, do too.

Another, fairly unusual, problem of the thirties is a particularly severe type of dandruff, which is actually a form of psoriasis. The flakes appear larger than normal dandruff, worse after shampooing and the scalp may suffer from irritable red patches. A shampoo containing coal extract should control the condition, but if it persists, consult an expert.

The Forties
During the forties the problems of ageing, which may have started to show in the thirties, become more prevalent – dry hair, dandruff, grey hair and hair that has lost its colour and life.

The dryness is caused by a further slowing down in the production of oil by the sebaceous glands and will usually be a problem in skin all over the body too. Use a rich shampoo for dry hair, leave hair conditioner on a little longer and give hair a deep conditioning treatment at least once a week. Dry hair naturally if possible or with a low heat to avoid loss of natural moisture.

Dandruff is usually the dry-scalp variety and dandruff shampoos are not necessarily the answer. Try a shampoo for dry hair, massaging the scalp as you lather; rinse thoroughly to cleanse the scalp of all loose flakes and, if this doesn't solve the problem, try alternating with a dandruff shampoo.

Grey hair can be disguised with products specially formulated to cover grey hair. Choose a colour near your natural colour for the best effect; better still, go to a professional colourist.

Dull hair means that the light is reflected evenly or not reflected at all and the hair looks drab and lifeless. A colour conditioning rinse, tint or sometimes henna will restore the lustre and gloss.

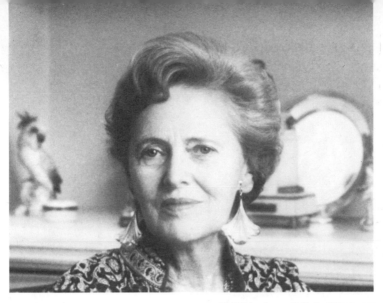

Fifty and Over

At this age most women have reached the menopause and, along with the other problems associated with this time, hair and scalp suffer from the change in hormonal balance that is occurring and the stress that is often present. The hair follicles are not receiving the support from hormones that they are used to and this may result in hair loss. Facial hair may coarsen or darken. Women receiving hormone treatment during menopause will probably find the hair fall less severe, but there is no reason why any woman should suffer distressing hair loss during menopause, providing she looks after her hair and scalp, cares for her body with proper diet and exercise and generally maintains her health.

Excessive hair fall, at any age, is something to take seriously, and professional advice should be sought. Dandruff at this time could be due to lack of circulation – massage, while the hair is being shampooed, will help, loosening scalp cells and stimulating blood flow. A soft hair style that doesn't need spraying into place, allows the hair to be brushed through and the scalp massaged between shampoos will also help this type of dandruff.

Greying hair will also become drier, needing a good rich shampoo and conditioner, and the scalp must be kept clean.

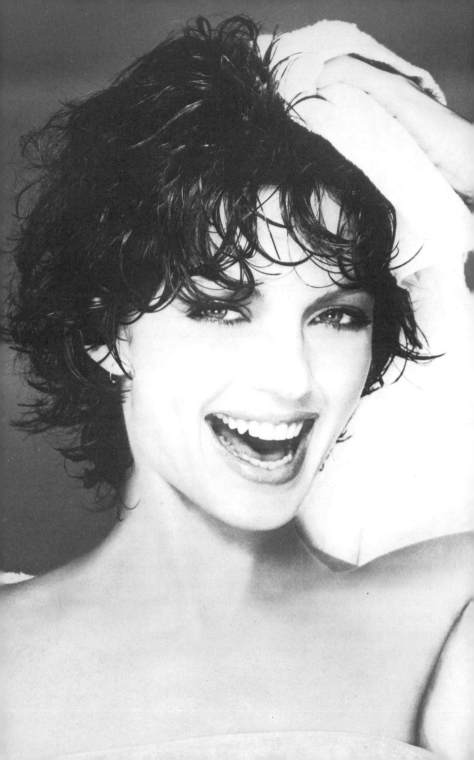

Hair Care

Healthy hair is always high on any list of important beauty assets. Correct hair-care routine is vital if it's to look its best all the time. How can you arrive at the correct routine for your hair? First, establish your hair type – is it oily, dry, mixed or normal? Then its texture – is it fine, medium or coarse? Is it thick or thin? Curly or straight? Choose products especially formulated for your hair type.

Shampooing
You can shampoo your hair every day if you like – twice a day if necessary. The modern rule is: wash whenever it looks or feels in need; the vital thing is to use a mild shampoo that is correctly formulated for your type of hair.

The key to healthy hair is a healthy scalp, which allows the hair follicles and the sebaceous glands attached to them to function efficiently. Don't scrub as you wash; treat your hair as gently as fabric and massage the scalp as you lather. Carelessness at this stage can harm your hair. A good method is to soak your hair first in warm water, then apply the shampoo. Don't use too much shampoo – many are very concentrated; it does no harm to dilute in a little water before applying – and make sure the shampoo is spread evenly through your hair. A good trick to ensure this is to pour it first into the palms of your hands, rub them together and then apply to your hair. You can always add more shampoo if you need it. Then rinse, rinse and rinse again – there is no point in spending hours styling your hair if it isn't clean when you start.

If you wash your hair very frequently you probably need only one application each time – too much shampoo too often will strip the hair shaft of all the natural oils it needs to provide the lustre and manageability you are looking for.

To find the right shampoo for your hair may take a little experimenting. First read the labels to find one that is designed for your kind of hair – they should tell you (apart from whether they are for oily, dry or balanced hair) whether they have a medicated ingredient for dandruff, are hypo-allergenic, have an additive to treat tinted or bleached hair, are enriched to control flyaway hair and whether they are based on natural or plant extracts. Many will refer to a pH factor – this is the measure of the liquid's acidity or alkalinity. Hair is surrounded by a liquid mantle of atmospheric moisture, perspiration and so forth. Ideally this liquid mantle should be slightly acidic. Many of the things we routinely do to hair, like colouring, permanent waving and straightening, even shampooing, can leave an alkaline residue. This alkalinity can weaken the hair's structure, making it less resilient or elastic and thus more prone to breaking and splitting. The pH products are aimed at maintaining the natural acid/alkaline balance of the hair's moisture mantle, but should only be necessary for chemically altered hair – i.e., that which has been coloured, bleached, permed or straightened.

Dry shampoos mostly come in powder form and are based on talc or cornstarch. The method is to shake a little into the hair, distribute it by rubbing gently so that it absorbs oil and dirt and then brush it out. Its best use is for people with oily hair and for fringes, which tend to become oily more quickly than the rest of the head. Alternatively, dabbing the scalp with an astringent lotion, witch-hazel or eau-de-Cologne will usually do the trick.

Conditioning

A conditioner for your hair is like a moisturizer for your skin – after cleansing you use a moisturizer, after shampooing you should use

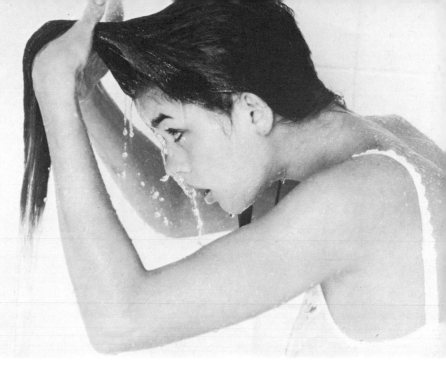

a conditioner. The purpose of a conditioner is to counteract dryness of the hair shaft, to smooth and make it manageable by making it easier to comb through and style and to help prevent split ends and breakage.

When you consider that any single strand of hair on your head can be as old as six years – which means six years of exposure to sun, wind, water, curling, brushing, styling and probably tinting, perming or straightening, it is no wonder it is no longer in its original healthy condition and needs all the help it can get.

The moment the hair appears on the scalp and leaves its follicle beneath the skin it ceases to receive nourishment from the papilla – the only help it gets is from the oil-glands attached to the follicle, which should provide enough oil to flow down the shaft and condition it. However, all abuses tend to strip the hair shaft of this natural lubrication and the ends especially become very dry and brittle.

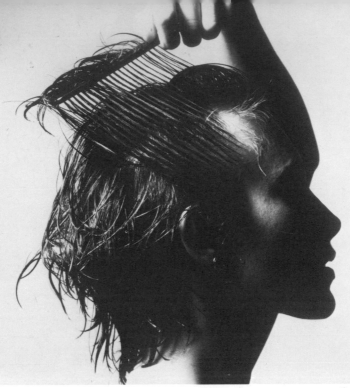

A conditioner is, therefore, a vital part of your hair-care routine if it's to stay healthy and glossy. There are instant conditioners and cream rinses to use each time you shampoo, and deep-penetrating conditioning treatments to use once or twice a week, if the hair is damaged or very dry; or once a month, for healthy maintenance.

After shampooing, hair has a negative electric charge, the degree of which depends on the humidity and the shampoo; it can be greater on some days than on others. It makes each hair strand stand away from its neighbour, causing flyaway hair, and conditioners compensate by adding a positive electric charge.

The method of applying conditioner is similar to shampooing except that you don't need to pre-rinse as the hair is already wet and pliable from rinsing off the shampoo. Use conditioners sparingly and start by putting a small amount in the palms of your

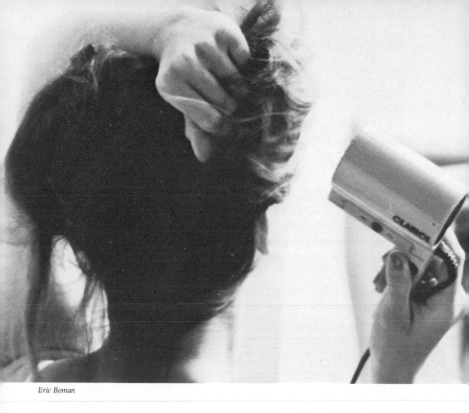

hands, rubbing them together and applying flat to your hair. Then, with your fingers, comb the conditioner through your hair and along the hair shafts and leave it on for a minute. Rinse off very thoroughly. Finish with a cold-water rinse, which helps make hair shinier because it closes the scales on the outer layer or cuticle of the hair shaft, making them all lie in one direction and thus providing a smoother surface.

Deep conditioning treatments are essential to restore damaged or dried-out hair at the end of a summer or winter sports holiday, or if the hair has been over-bleached or tinted or badly permed. Some – particularly home-made conditioners containing olive, nut or light vegetable oils – are applied before shampooing, preferably the night before; others are applied afterwards and left on between ten and thirty minutes before being rinsed out.

Recipes for Shampoos and Conditioners

Shampoo

Try the oldest shampoo of all – the herb saponaria or soapwort. You can buy the dried root in packets (it is often used to clean old and delicate fabrics).

Put 0·9 oz. (25 g) of saponaria with $1\frac{3}{4}$ pints (1 litre) of water into a non-aluminium pan, bring to the boil, then simmer for 20 minutes, stirring occasionally. Let it stand until cool, then strain through muslin. Make up the liquid to $1\frac{3}{4}$ pints (1 litre) with a strong infusion of another herb such as camomile (for fair hair), rosemary (for dark hair) or nettle (for scalp problems).

Conditioner

Mashed avocado or beaten eggs work wonders on dull lifeless hair – leave on for 15–20 minutes, then rinse well – but probably the best home hair treatment of all is warm oil.

Heat a small amount of olive oil, or any good vegetable oil, to blood temperature. About $\frac{1}{4}$ pint (0·14 litres) should be enough. Apply it to the scalp by parting the hair in sections, until the whole head is thoroughly saturated, then comb through with a wide-toothed comb and massage the scalp. Finally wrap the head in tinfoil or a plastic cap and cover with a warm towel. Leave on overnight if possible, then wash twice with a good mild shampoo and rinse thoroughly.

Rinse

To help hair shine and keep the scalp healthy, make a final rinse from the juice of a fresh lemon diluted in really cold water – this closes the pores on the scalp and makes the overlapping scales on the hair shaft lie flat and reflect the light.

Quick pick-ups

Powdered orris root is a natural dry shampoo; the hair should be divided in sections and the powder scattered down the partings. Leave for five minutes, then brush out thoroughly. A good tip is to cover the brush with a piece of absorbent fabric (muslin, gauze or nylon) sprinkled with a mild astringent like witch-hazel or eau-de-

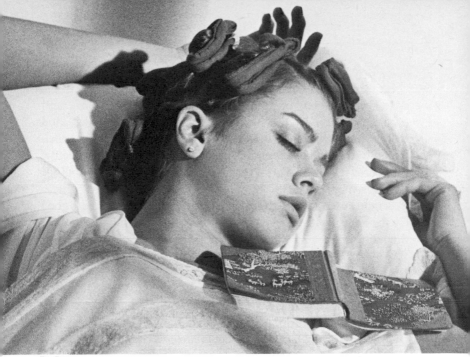

Eric Boman

Cologne – this will help remove grease and dust and speed up the process of removing the powder.

Alternatively the astringent alone can be massaged into the scalp down the partings – this will act as a temporary dry-clean and is useful if someone is bedridden and cannot move their head.

Brushing and Combing

In the days when there were no such things as conditioners and ladies had waist-length hair, there might have been some sense in the old rule: 'brush a hundred strokes a day'. But today excessive brushing can put such stress on hair that it splits, breaks or comes out at the roots, especially if it has been chemically altered or is very dry. Brushing also spreads scalp conditions, dirt and debris, so if you like to do it, the brush itself must be kept absolutely clean. Only brush hair when it is absolutely dry – wet hair is particularly vulnerable to breakage from brushing.

As a general rule, combing is best, but if brushing is vital to the style, keep it to a minimum and finish putting the hair in place with a comb. Always let the hair cool before removing rollers and remove the bottom ones first to avoid tangling the hair; then brush or comb straight back, but gently, to distribute the waves evenly. Don't drag it or you will run the risk of pulling it out by the roots or breaking the strands.

Bending over and brushing from the nape to the forehead is good for the scalp, as it stimulates circulation, and also adds fullness to the hair.

Drying

After shampooing and conditioning, the next step in hair care is drying. As much damage can be caused at this stage as any other and it is important to dry your hair the right way. The best way is to let it dry naturally, but many people haven't the time for this, so this is the next best method.

First blot out excess water with a towel. Then comb hair through using a wide-toothed comb, starting at the ends and working towards the scalp, removing tangles as you go. With another dry towel blot out any further moisture by wrapping it smoothly around your head and squeezing it around the ends. Then set and blow-dry or sit under the drier. Don't over-dry – if you can find the time, let the heated air cool off; then dry naturally for the last few minutes. This will prevent any danger of the hair shaft drying out and being damaged.

Blow-drying must be done with care to avoid the hair tangling and breaking off. Divide it into sections and, as you dry, lift each section of hair up and away from the scalp and wrap round a brush. Plastic ones with widely spaced, soft, elastic bristles are best. Now blow the section dry, working from the root to the end of the strands. Start at the back, at the nape of the neck (pin the rest of the hair on top of your head to get it out of the way), work around the sides, around the face and lastly dry the crown.

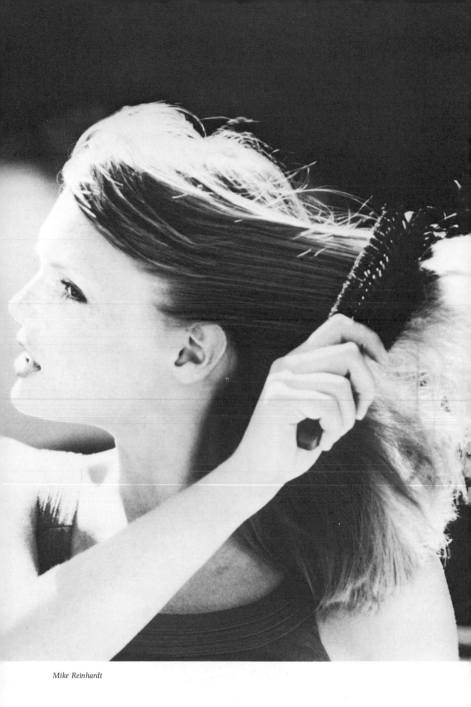

Mike Reinhardt

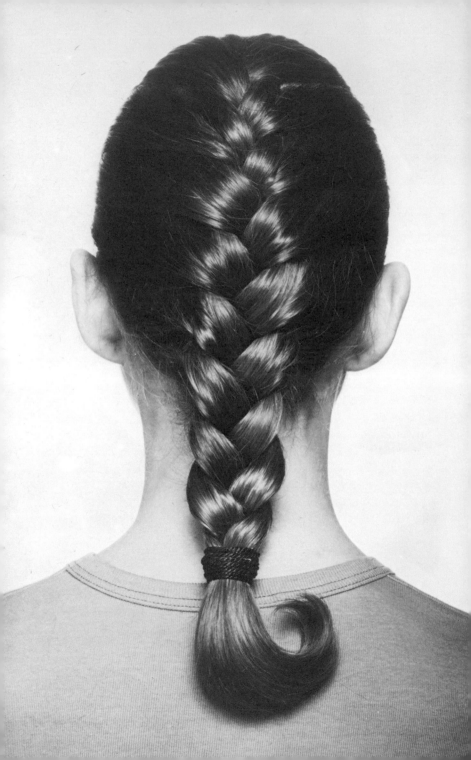

Hair Styles

One of the most important things to know about your hair is its limitations. Learn to live with them. This means accepting your hair's texture. If it is fine, it probably tends to be flyaway and doesn't hold a set well. If it's medium, it probably behaves itself quite well and holds a set. If it's coarse, it is probably unruly and hard to curl. It also means accepting the amount of hair you have – its body or bulk. If the hairs on your head are massed and close together, your hair is thick. If they're sparse, your hair is thin. The amount of straightness or curliness imposes some limitations, though perming or straightening can usually correct this. You are born with these qualities and there is nothing you can do to change them, so make the best of them. Fine hair is usually thin and looks fullest and best when it's blunt-cut and not much longer than chin length. Medium-textured hair with medium body can take almost any kind of style or length – it has the fewest limitations. Coarse hair often responds well to a longish blunt-cut. The length tends to weight the hair down and make it behave. Too short a cut is apt to leave you with hair that bushes and sticks out.

If hair is curly, humidity will make it curl more. Chemical straightening can be a solution, if you insist on a straight look.

Straight hair, especially if it's fine, will usually resist curling except under good weather conditions. So again, your best plan is to find a style that doesn't rely too much on curl, unless you invest in a good permanent wave. This, depending on how fast your hair grows, is a fairly temporary solution and can be expensive if your hair needs re-perming often. However, modern soft perms are very good indeed and do offer the straight-haired person the chance of a complete change of look.

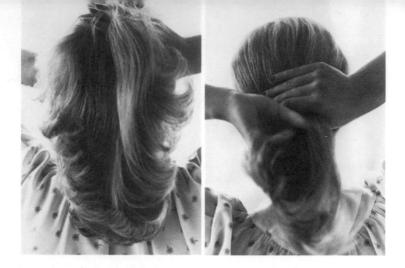

How to Make a Top Knot

1. *Hair must be long enough to scoop up off the face, without leaving too many loose strands. Beforehand, brush hair forward to give it body and then smoothly back off the face.* **2.** *Take all the hair from above the ears and around the face up to the crown and hold it while the back section is combed in to join it.* **3.** *Hold the hair tightly in place where the finished knot will be, twist it until it coils around neatly and the ends can be tucked in.* **4.** *Finally secure the knot with grips or ornamental hairpins.* **5.** OPPOSITE *The finished effect: a neat small head, cool and comfortable for summer.*

Sandra Lousada

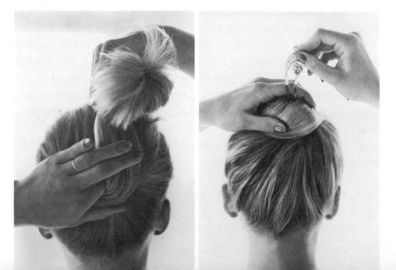

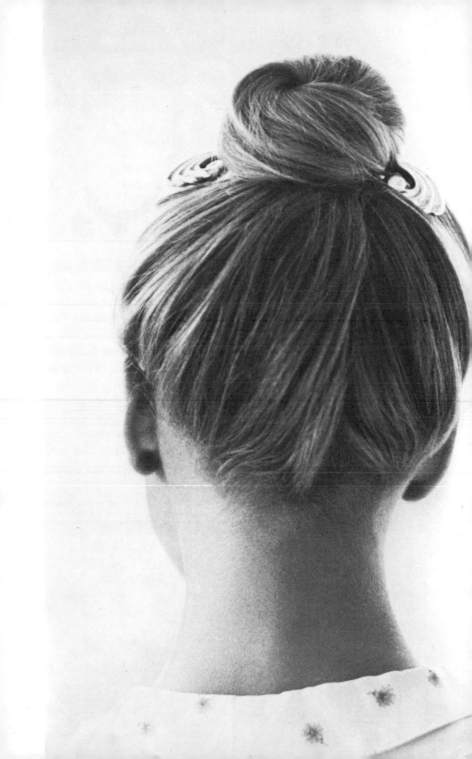

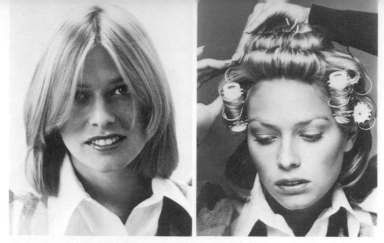

Blow-Drying and Rollers

1. *With this good basic cut, several things can be done: it can be blow-dried for a sleek, barely curved look; set with heated rollers for the curly look, or with a combination of regular rollers and a hand drier for a long-lasting pageboy.* **2.** *For the curly look: Blow-dry the hair, not to style it but just to dry and smooth it. Then set with medium-sized rollers, two on top, three on each side, two turned under, one close to the face rolled forward. The back is set in one row of large rollers rolled to the nape. When the rollers have cooled, unroll them, brush hair gently into shape. For extra hold try one of the wetting-plus-conditioner products made especially for use with heated rollers.* **3.** *For the pageboy: For more hold than just a blow-dry will give, use a large regular roller clipped to the scalp on either side and two in the back. Let blow-drier heat set them for a minute or two.* **4.** *For added fullness on top use four rollers, and two pin curls for the shorter side.* **5.** OPPOSITE *The soft, curly look.*

Mike Reinhardt

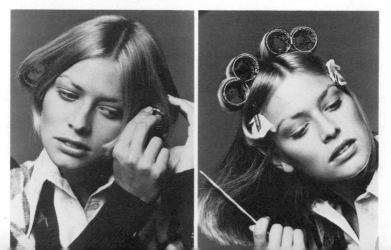

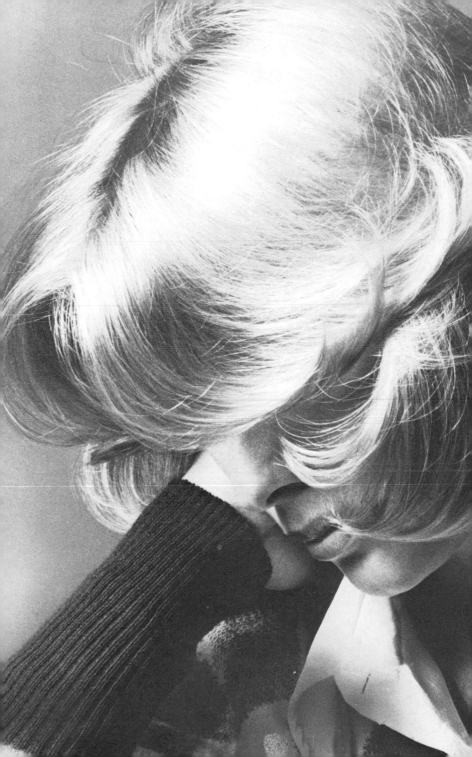

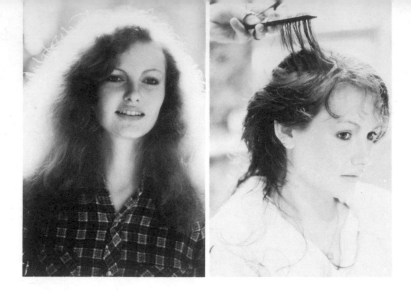

Cutting your Hair from Long to Short

1. *The change cutting makes can be dramatic, as it is here: from shoulder length to three-inch layer at the back with shorter hair in front. This looks even shorter as the model's hair is also naturally curly.* **2.** *After shampooing, the hair is cut in sections from front to back so that it can be seen how the new shape suits the model's face, and if necessary be adjusted. The length at the sides is carefully watched so that the hair does*

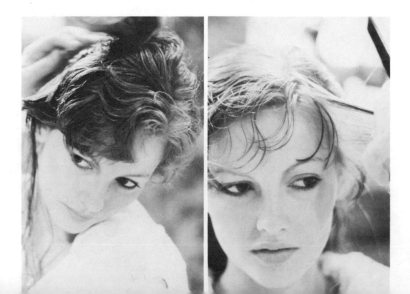

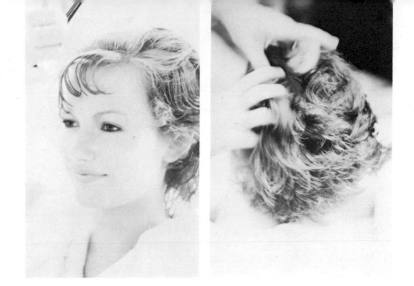

not get pushed up by ears. 3. *Halfway through the cutting it is already apparent how flattering this style is to the model's face.* 4. *The hair is kept wet while cutting.* 5. *The hair continues to be cut in sections, as the nape is neared.* 6. *An anti-static and light setting lotion is rubbed through, and the hair is towelled dry.* 7. *It is finally finger dried, and when completely dry the roots are sprayed again to bring out the curl and left to dry naturally into the finished shape.* 8. *The dramatic result.*

Sandra Lousada

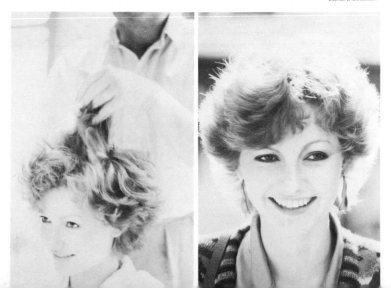

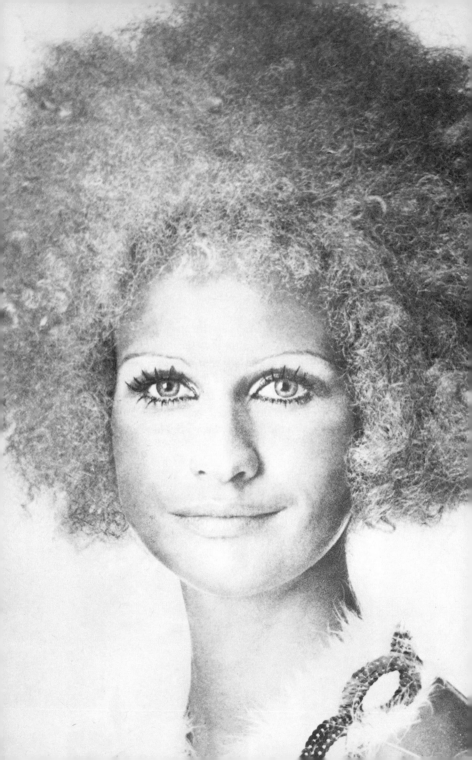

Glossary of Recent Cuts and Styles

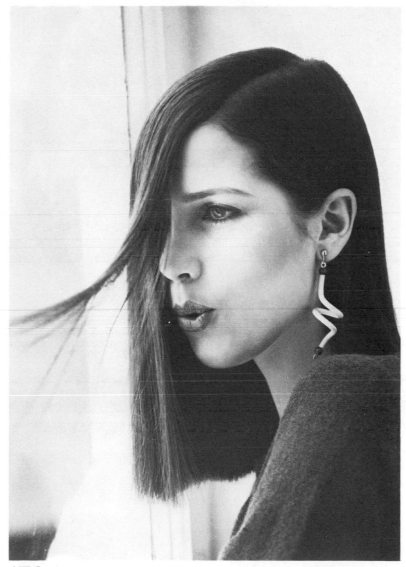

◁ AFRO *Penn*

BLUNT *Sandra Lousada*

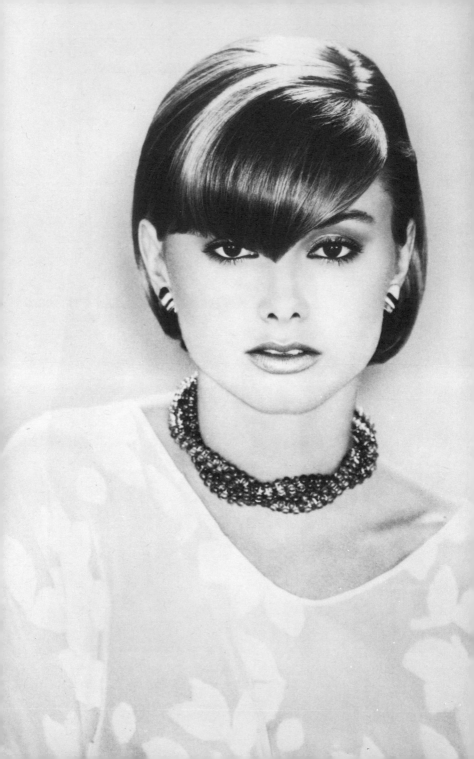

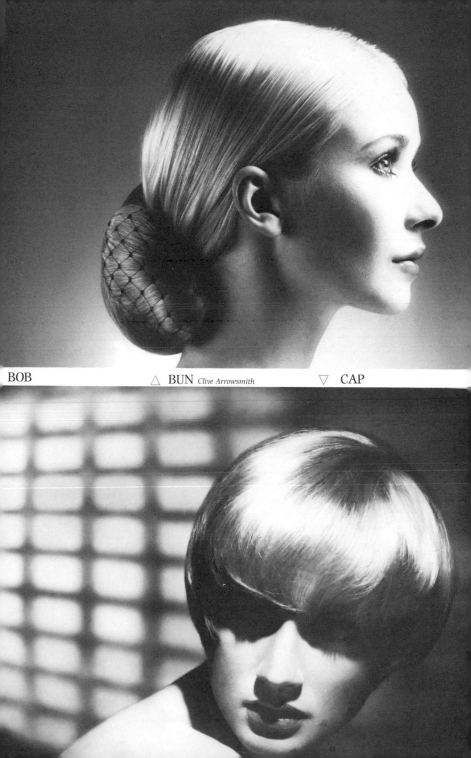

BOB   △ BUN *Clive Arrowsmith*   ▽ CAP

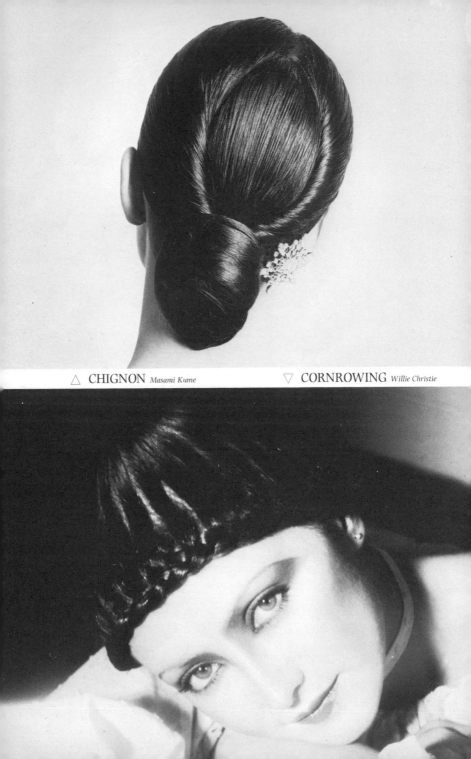

△ CHIGNON *Masami Kume*   ▽ CORNROWING *Willie Christie*

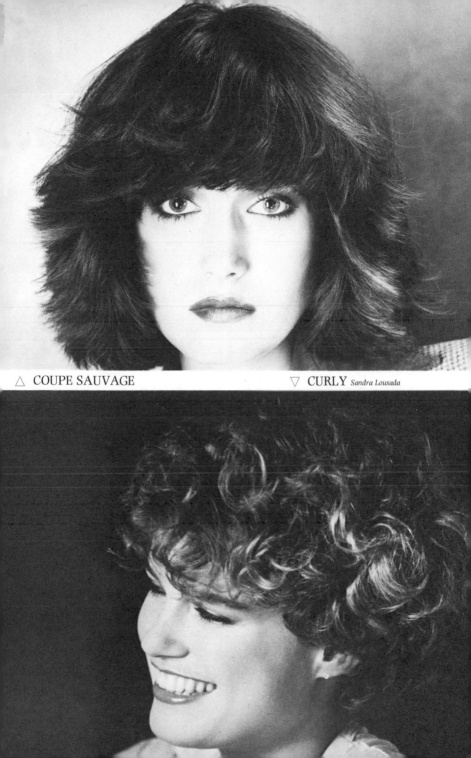

△ COUPE SAUVAGE ▽ CURLY *Sandra Lousada*

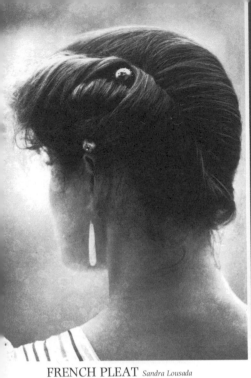

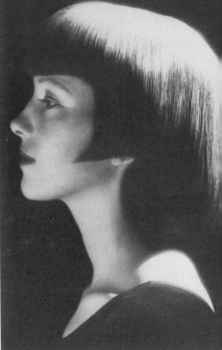

FRENCH PLEAT *Sandra Lousada*
GEORGE *Mike Reinhardt*

GEOMETRIC *Sandra Lousada*
LAYERED LONG

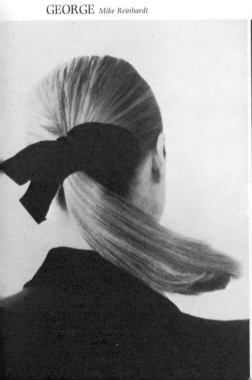

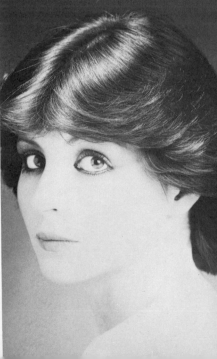

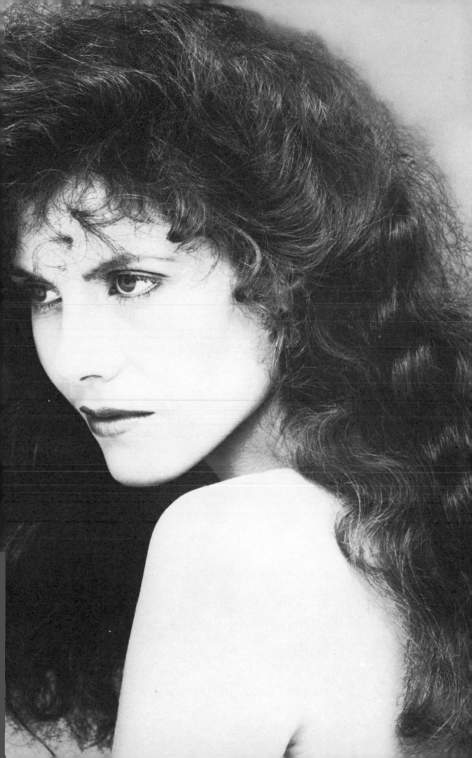

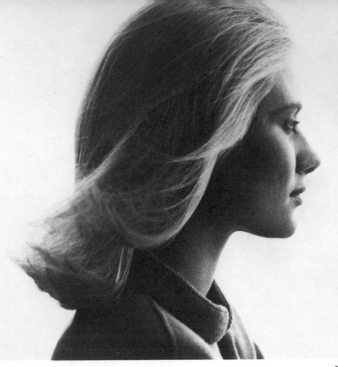

MEDIUM *Sandra Lousada*
PAGEBOY

PLAITS *Fouli Elia*

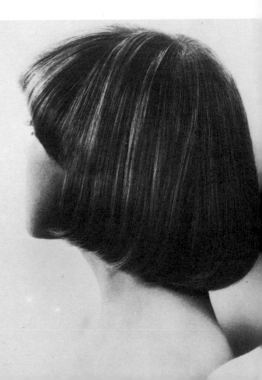

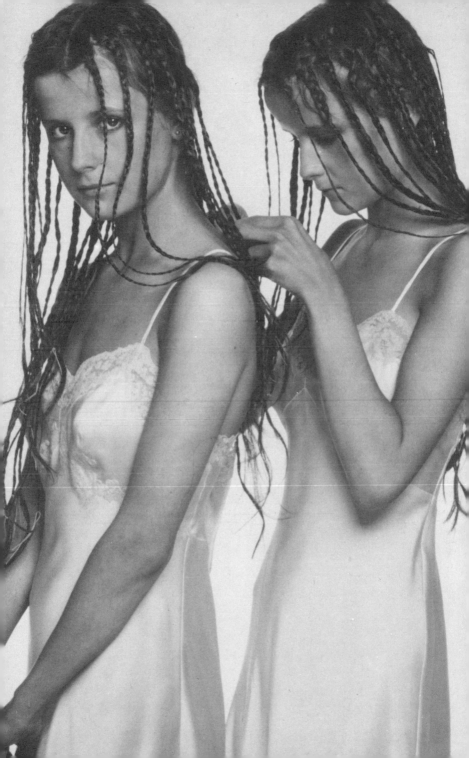

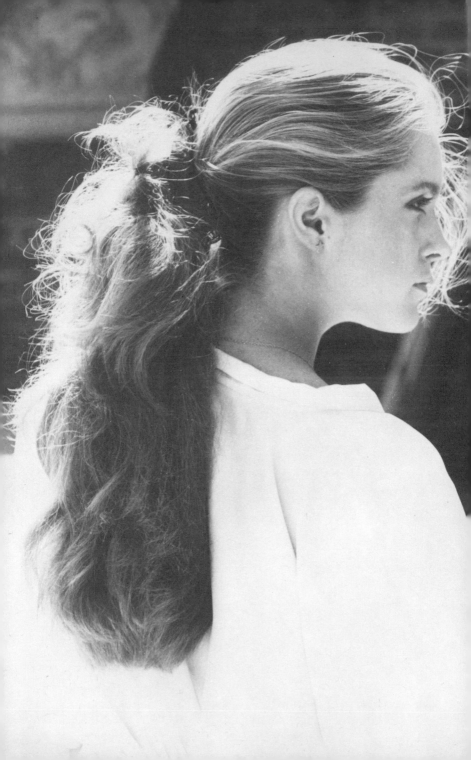

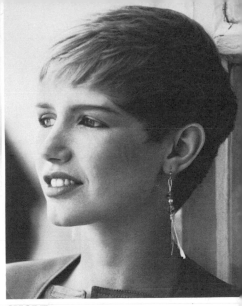

◁ PONYTAIL *Sandra Lousada*
△ PUNK *Masami Kume*

SHORT *Sandra Lousada*
STRAIGHT

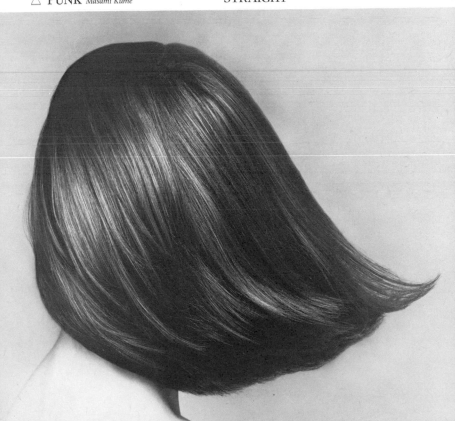

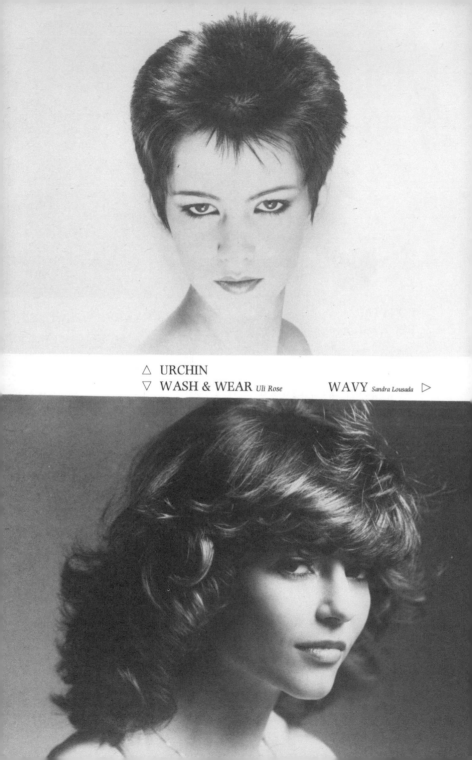

△ URCHIN
▽ WASH & WEAR *Uli Rose*   WAVY *Sandra Lousada* ▷

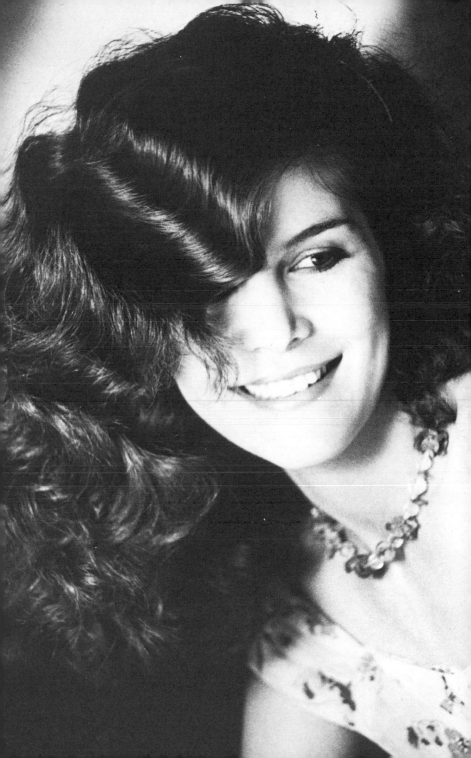

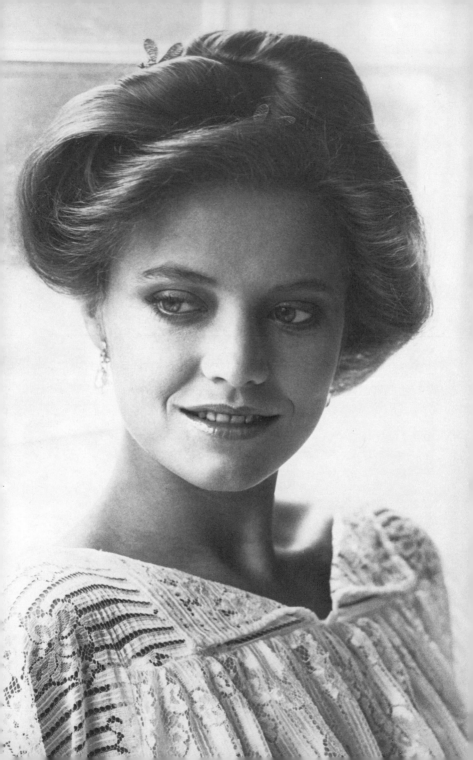

Special Occasions: Style and Decoration

Many people make the mistake of changing their hair style for a special occasion so drastically that their family and friends hardly recognize them – that's fine if the new style is an improvement, but often it's done with no forethought as to whether it suits them or not. It is vital to try out the transformation you have in mind before the actual moment of wearing it.

Effects can often be achieved for an occasion or a photograph that wouldn't be possible on a daily basis, e.g., hair that's too short to 'go up' can be coaxed over padding or have a piece added, but it is costly, as it takes time and expertise. Equally, long hair can be made to look short; this is easier as it can be wrapped, plaited, twisted or folded away, giving the effect of a tiny head. And, the back is all-important.

Many styles totally unsuited to modern daily life still look wonderful with a wedding or ball dress, but only on those occasions; for that, a good hairdresser will want to know what kind of head-dress, hat or veil is going to be worn, they will also want to know what jewellery, if any, is going to be worn and the design of the dress before suggesting a hair style.

Particularly for weddings, it is a good idea to have a complete dress rehearsal, if possible, as no one wants to be worried that their hair will fall down under the weight of an antique lace veil, or that the head-dress or decoration will not be secured firmly enough if there is a sudden gust of wind.

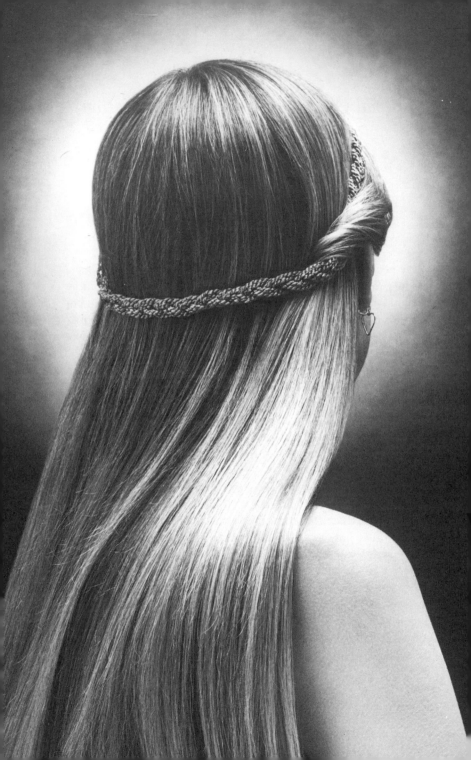

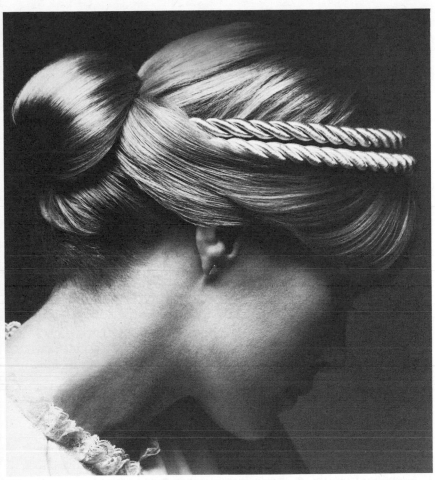

Ulli Rose

Special Occasions: Style and Decoration

John Swannell

Wigs and Hairpieces

Wigs have been in existence for centuries – the ancient Egyptians, Greeks and Romans wore them, Elizabeth I had over eighty and throughout history they have played an important part in fashion.

Today, they are much in demand as a holiday accessory – to cover hair if it doesn't look too good after a day in the sun or in water; as an amusing part of the fashion scene, in brilliant colours far removed from natural hair; and as a cover-up for people with hair problems, from limp, oily, fine hair to complete baldness. Provided that they fit properly and are well styled, they are lightweight, easy to wear and less and less obviously wigs. They have another use too – they are an excellent way to try out a new hair style. Before cutting off all your hair or spending months growing it, try on a wig and see if the style really suits you.

There are two ways to buy a wig now – they can still be ordered, made-to-measure and probably of real hair, from your hairdresser. These are hand-made and obviously fit better and are therefore the most satisfactory, but they are also expensive and need professional cleaning and setting by a hairdresser. The alternative is to choose from the vast selection of ready-made wigs available at hairdressers and most department stores. Most of these are made from synthetic fibres, which have the advantage of being able to withstand rain, sleet, snow and humidity (one of the arch-enemies of hair). And when you wash them there's no need to worry about setting as they will revert to their original shape as they dry. They need minimal care, but between washes and when they're not being worn, they can be hung on a doorknob, turned inside out for airing, or stored in a box wrapped in tissue paper. They shouldn't be squashed or near too much heat. Give the wig a good brush or comb through every two or three days and shampoo regularly. Swish through in cool suds, rinse in cold water and drip-dry on a wig block if possible.

When you try on a wig you must take time to get it on properly. Ideally your own hair should be pinned in flat curls so that there is nothing to interfere with the shape of the wig and so you don't upset the angle by tucking in loose strands of your own hair. Put a wig on from the front, holding it firm on the forehead (it's easier if you get a friend to help the first time) while you ease it down on both sides and at the back. Then adjust it to fit securely – it should be firm but not tight, and you can always secure it on the crown with hairpins if necessary. Unless the style has a fringe, it is a good idea to fit the wig half an inch or so back from your face, then blend in your own hair over the edge of the wig. When you wear a wig it's rather like a close-fitting hat – the scalp heat is enclosed, the glands start producing more oil and the pores sweat. Therefore, if you suffer from any scalp disorder such as dandruff, it will become worse; also, your hair will quickly become lank, even if it was clean when you put the wig on. Because of this build-up of heat, it is vital to keep your hair and scalp clean – wash it daily if you are wearing a wig every day – and to wash or clean the wig regularly too. A dirty wig will spread infection very quickly. However often you wear a wig, you must give your scalp time to breathe. Prolonged covering by a wig can cause hair loss and scalp disorders.

Extra pieces or falls of hair are marvellous for occasional use, to increase the volume of the hair or add to a chignon, for instance. But because they have to be pinned very tightly to the real hair, they are potentially more damaging than wigs and should be used as rarely as possible. Hairpieces made of synthetic fibre are as satisfactory as real hair and can be cared for at home in the same way as wigs; those made by hand out of real hair need professional cleaning and styling by a hairdresser.

You and Your Hairdresser

The key to being happy with the way your hair looks is a good relationship with your hairdresser. However brilliant a hairdresser is – or you think he or she must be from seeing pictures of their work in newspapers and magazines – it is rare that you will obtain the perfect style the first time you visit the salon, although they will surely do their very best to make a new client happy and give the best possible cut.

Very often it is only after they have done your hair for several weeks, re-cut it, styled it for everyday and special occasions, seen (and heard from you) how it behaves away from their care, that you and they will begin to understand what is best for you and your hair. You must build up an atmosphere of mutual trust – you can expect thorough shampooing, advice on conditioning, colouring, permanent waving, straightening and all aspects of hair style and care. In return they need to learn how much time you devote to looking after your hair, how good you are at doing it yourself, what kind of life you lead, whether you eat and drink sensibly, sleep enough, exercise enough – in fact how much you really care about your looks generally. In time, you will learn to live with the hair you have and your hairdresser will teach you not to force your hair into shapes it cannot hold but to be happy if it's in the best possible condition and behaving as well as it possibly can. These days few women go daily to a hairdresser for a 'comb-out' or even regularly for a shampoo and set; the modern approach is to go once every four or five weeks for a cut, regularly for a conditioning treatment, whenever it is necessary to adjust or change the colour – and occasionally for a special event. A regular cut is one of the best beauty investments you can make – it keeps hair in shape, ensures that the ends don't dry out and split and makes it as easy as possible to look after at home. A professional conditioning treatment is also worthwhile – even women who have cared for their hair properly all their lives find that the condition sometimes deteriorates as a result of sickness (and intake of drugs), the stress of long-distance travel, climatic variations and over-exposure to the elements, or over-use of electrical aids like hair-driers and heated rollers; for them, a deep conditioning treatment at a salon can be of enormous benefit.

Clients should listen carefully to their hairdressers' advice before rushing headlong into a new cut, perm or drastic change of colour – the chances are that what they've got in mind has nothing to do with what would be successful with their type of hair or what would suit them; a good hairdresser will be able to suggest changes that *are* possible, and *will* suit them, and will therefore give them the new look and change they crave.

An expert hairdresser never stops learning from his clients – using their experiences to help others with similar situations or problems. A jet-setter, for instance, whom he sees regularly, although perhaps only every six months, is usually full of tips and tales on how to cope with hair in whatever climate and place she's just visited – and whether local hairdressers are good, bad or indifferent, whether she wished her hair had been a different length or whether it was just right for once: information invaluable to the next client, who is just off to that part of the world. A mother (who is a long-standing client) may bring in a teenage daughter who needs persuading that she'll regret a hard, geometric cut with her pretty, soft features – and a clever hairdresser who has known her, or about her, will succeed in giving her a cut to make everyone happy.

Permanent Waving and Straightening

Perming and straightening, even more than colouring, are potentially dangerous to the hair's health, because they alter the basic, natural structure of the hair shaft. It is absolutely vital that the processes are done with immense care and great expertise. When hair is wet it is in a relaxed, pliable state and can sometimes be stretched to as much as one third more than its original length before breaking – but it shrinks as it dries and will have returned to normal length by the time it is completely dry.

If you want to curl it temporarily, it is necessary to wet or dampen it and wind it round rollers or pipe-cleaners, tie it in rags or secure it in flat pin curls. When it has dried, the hair will be curly and remain so until wetted again – either intentionally or in a rainstorm, a humid climate or a steamy bathroom. Wet hair is obviously very vulnerable to breakage – which is why it should never be brushed – and should be treated with the greatest care and just coaxed into shape. The alternative to this method is to use heated rollers, which force the hair to accept a new direction, but the curl will still fall out when it becomes wet or damp. The disadvantage of this method is that it dries out the ends of the hair shaft, but it is very convenient. Permanent waving takes the temporary curling process a huge step further by *sealing* the shaft's new direction with the aid of chemicals, so that it doesn't disappear the next time the hair is soaked. These chemicals penetrate the cuticle of the hair shaft, enter the cortex and alter the natural line of the hair to a soft wave or tight curl, depending on the size of the roller the hair is wrapped around when the perm solution is applied. A soft, wavy result is often called a body wave, medium curls a straightforward perm and the frizzy variety an 'Afro', but they are all achieved by the process of permanent waving and will grow out as the hair grows from the roots and the ends are cut off. The danger of permanent waving lies in timing. Whether the perm is done at home or in a salon, precise timing is essential if the hair is not to be damaged by over-processing. This means that it can be literally dissolved by leaving the perm solution on too long, break off at the roots or become over-dry, not only at the ends but right down the hair shaft. Total concentration is required from the person doing the perm – kitchen timers are very useful to make sure the process is stopped at the appropriate moment. If perming at home is chosen, read every word of the manufacturers' instructions and follow them in every detail. No hair should be permed more often than every three or four months; if tinted, it should not be permed within two weeks either way of the colouring process; and hair that is in any way damaged already should not be permed at all.

Straightening is probably the most drastic thing that can be done to hair – it employs the perming process in reverse, i.e., instead of allowing the hair to shrink into a sealed wave, it stretches the hair straight and seals that straightness.

Because hair breaks even more easily when wet and stretched, straightening must only be done by an expert and only on hair that is strong enough in both texture and condition to take the strong chemicals employed. Instead of winding the hair round rollers when the perm solution is applied, the hair is gently combed straight from as close to the roots as possible, relaxing it and easing it into straightness. This combing must continue until the desired shape is achieved and the solution rinsed off.

The result will last until the hair is cut, but the straight effect will be reduced as the new hair shafts grow naturally curly from the root. Straightening is therefore not so successful as perming from a long-term point of view.

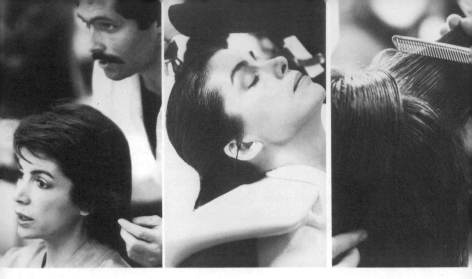

Straight to Curly: Perming your Hair

1. *The author discusses her cut and shape with her hairdresser.* **2.** *Pre-perm shampoo and conditioning.* **3.** *Hair cut: volume removed with reverse layering technique – starting at the front with straight fringe to get the right length, and not have it fall too heavily or square on top – and moving straight to the back, leaving the longest hair behind the ears and at the nape.* **4.** *Hair examined for texture, correct perming lotion chosen.* **5.** *Hair curled section by section, using the normal method with curling rods and papers.* **6.** *Hair curled from the front backwards, as*

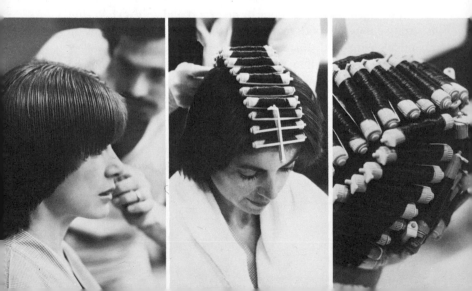

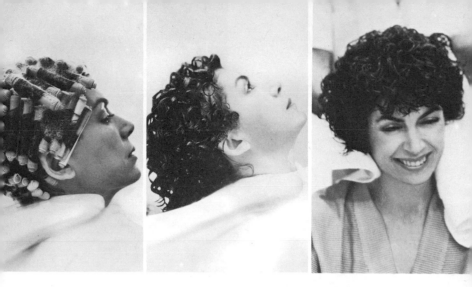

hair is to move back off the face. **7.** Forty minutes later, over to the backwash for ten minutes of neutralizing with the curlers in. **8.** Five minutes more with curlers removed and hair loose. **9.** After thorough rinse and condition, hair rough-dried with towel. **10.** Dried with Air-Stop attachment on a hand drier to avoid static electricity, and give maximum body. **11.** While being dried, hair is shaped with fingers. **12.** A completely new look, as hair is lifted away from the face, the perm giving it body and movement.

Sandra Lousada

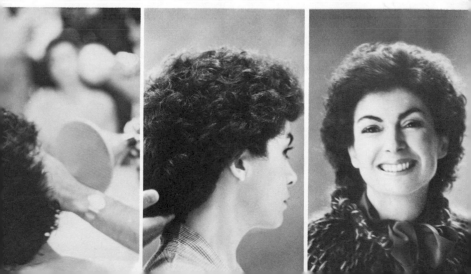

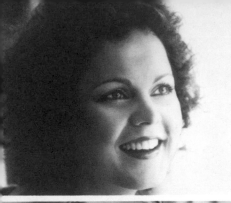
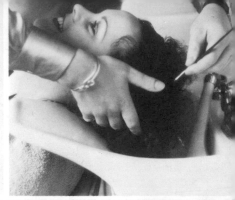
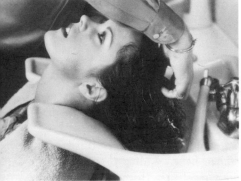
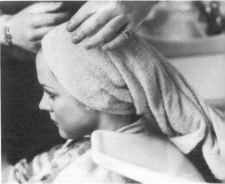
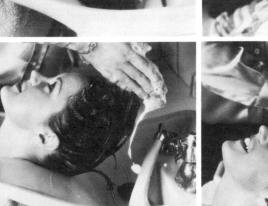
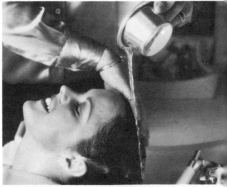
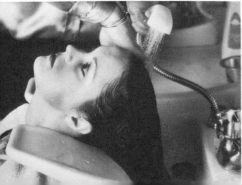
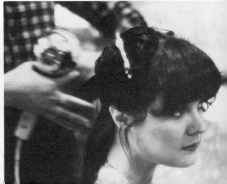

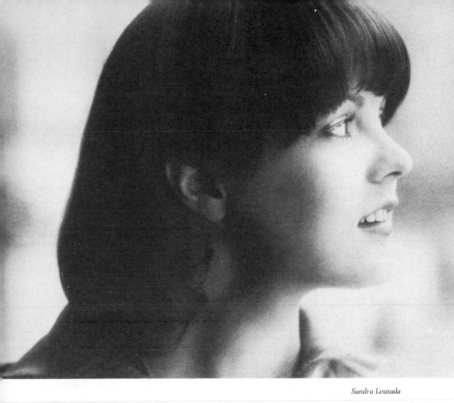

Curly to Straight

1. OPPOSITE, TOP LEFT *Model's hair in its natural state, curling tightly back from the face.* **2.** OPPOSITE, TOP RIGHT *The hair is to be straightened: first a 'relaxer' cream is painted onto the hair, with a brush.* **3.** *The cream is combed carefully through, and the hair is wrapped in a towel to warm the relaxing process.* **4.** *The hair is thoroughly shampooed.* **5.** *Then neutralised for ten minutes.* **6 and 7.** *Finally it is thoroughly conditioned and rinsed.* **8.** *Hair is blow dried.* **9.** ABOVE *The new straightened hair looks thicker and a richer brown, because the light was not getting through the curls. It also lengthened out to a head of hair to the shoulders with a full fringe.*

An A–Z of Hair Health

Allergies

Allergies resulting in a rash on the skin can appear on the scalp as easily as anywhere else on the body. Identifying the cause is often difficult, as there are hundreds of known, and many unknown, allergens. Use a mild shampoo as often as necessary and try not to aggravate the condition by scratching.

Alopecia

Alopecia areata, Alopecia totalis, traction Alopecia and banded Alopecia are various kinds of hair loss. *Alopecia areata* is loss of hair in patches and can develop into *Alopecia totalis*, or complete baldness. *Traction* and *banded Alopecia* result from an intolerable strain being put on the hair – from being pulled back into a tight ponytail or being pulled as it is straightened – and usually occur around the hairline. If this pressure is removed there is every chance the hair will regrow, but if the abuse continues the hair loss may be permanent.

Anaemia

Of the various varieties of anaemia, those caused by poor diet, lack of iron or vitamin deficiency (particularly vitamin B) will most affect the hair. Once the condition is halted, treated, and the diet improved, hair too will gradually return to health.

Bad Hair Odour

This usually occurs in conjuction with excessively oily hair conditions. It is the result of sweat- and oil-glands overproducing, often because of stress, exhaustion and a diet too rich in oily and fried foods. Once the diet is corrected, the oily hair condition treated and the stress alleviated, the odour will disappear.

Baldness

Baldness, or Alopecia totalis, occurs when the hair follicles atrophy and cease to produce new hair. It usually begins with a thinning of the hair at the temples and crown, becoming more severe until only the sides and back of the head have any hair at all – and sometimes not even these areas are covered. Baldness is often hereditary; it used to be thought peculiar to men, but nowadays many women suffer from it – reinforcing the theory that frequently it is caused by stress and strain and is also sometimes the result of illness or drugs.

Cortisone

This very powerful drug has many side effects; among them are distressing hair loss on the head and the reverse: growth of facial hair. The best answer for the former is a wig – there are such good ones available now in so many colours and styles that they can do wonders for the morale. As for the latter, if the facial hair isn't too coarse or dark, try a facial hair bleach or a depilatory cream especially formulated for facial hair.

Dandruff

This term is used widely to describe any scaly condition of the scalp. It is often thought to be the result of a dry scalp, and this can be so, but more often it goes hand in hand with oily hair when the sebaceous glands are over-producing and the follicles get blocked. Causes include lack of fresh air or air circulation, i.e., if wigs are worn constantly or the head is often wrapped in scarves or covered with a hat; stress and emotional strain; and sudden changes in climate or diet. The scalp should be kept immaculately clean by frequent washing. Many anti-dandruff shampoos contain harsh ingredients, so it is sometimes suggested that a mild shampoo should be used alternately every other day with an anti-dandruff treatment. In other words, treat the condition with great gentleness: don't rub too hard or use anything too strong; wash frequently and rinse very thoroughly.

Dermatitis
This inflammation of the skin or scalp is also known as eczema.

Discoid Lupus Erythematosis
Related to dandruff, this condition appears as reddish-brown scaly patches with thinning hair in the centre and needs help from a doctor or dermatologist.

Drugs
Many medicines, even mild ones if taken over a long period of time, but particularly powerful modern drugs, cause the hair condition to change, the scalp to develop problems, or hair loss. If it is not possible to stop the medication, extra care must be taken over what food is eaten; shampoo and condition to keep the hair as healthy as possible; often vitamin supplements such as Brewers' Yeast tablets will help.

Dry Hair
Dry hair appears dull and brittle and is often caused by over-bleaching, perming or over-exposure to sun, wind, salt or chlorine-filled water. See also pages 95–6.

Eczema
This is a scalp disorder, also known as dermatitis, which is usually a reddish inflammation with damp, sometimes oozing, scales and which requires urgent attention from a doctor, dermatologist or trichologist.

Favus
This is a deep-rooted fungal infection, sometimes the result of ringworm left untreated for too long, affecting the scalp and sometimes the nails. It appears as yellow cup-like crusts, which stick together, then drop off, leaving the scalp hairless and scarred. Immediate attention from a doctor is essential.

Grey Hair
Grey hair, correctly defined, is hair where white hairs are mixed with the natural colour, giving a grey effect. If hair strands contain melanin (colour granules), they are 'coloured'; if they don't, they are 'white'. As the body ages, the hair bulbs fail to produce melanin in the hair shaft and white hair results. See also pages 103–4.

Hair Breakage
Hair usually breaks only when it is dry and brittle and this comes from abuse: over-processing by means of bleach, colour or permanent waves or over-exposure to the elements. Hair that is breaking is very fragile and needs the gentlest treatment to restore it to health; it should be combed gently with a wide-toothed comb, shampooed with a richer formula than usual and conditioned every time it is washed. Don't blow-dry or use heated rollers or other electric aids until it has returned to health – and only with the greatest caution even then.

Hair Fall
A hair that has fallen has a tiny white bulb at one end. Fifty to a hundred hairs falling out daily is normal – hair loss over and above that needs treatment. The causes are not all known but include contraceptive pills, chemotherapy, drugs like cortisone, anything that interferes with hormones, and emotional disorders such as anxiety, lack of sleep or tension. Finding the cause will determine how permanent the loss will be – often the excessive fall can be halted and the hair will regrow in time.

Hormones
Hormones affect the hair – a proper balance must be maintained or problems may arise. Hormones are used to treat baldness in men, but the side effects may be unattractive and the results uncertain.

Ichthyosis
This is a hereditary condition where the skin is abnormally dry and scaly – hence its other name, Fish Skin. If it appears on the scalp, it will mean the hair becomes so dry and fragile it cannot grow to any length and will break off in clumps. It needs medical attention and frequent washing with a mild shampoo to keep the scalp clean.

Lice
Lice, even today, are quite common, usually among schoolchildren. A child with lice in the hair will probably complain of an itching scalp and scratch it excessively. Examine the scalp under a good light, paying particular attention to the hairline; if moving lice or eggs are visible, immediate medical attention is required. A doctor will prescribe an anti-louse shampoo, which should be applied by an adult who will see it is used correctly.

Menopause
At this stage in women's lives, when menstruation ceases, the hormone balance is changing and can cause hair loss and neurodermatitis, a patchy form of dandruff.

Menstruation
The menstrual cycle affects the sebaceous glands and the amount of oil they produce; consequently, many women find their hair oilier at the beginning and end of their period.

Mixed Condition Hair
Mixed condition hair appears as an oily scalp and dry hair. See also pages 96–7.

Neurodermatitis
This is usually a clearly defined patch of really heavy dandruff-like scales at the nape of the neck, and is very itchy. The scalp next to it is quite often clean and healthy, but the patch needs urgent treatment. This condition is most prevalent among older women, often appearing during the menopause and after.

Oily Hair
Oily hair becomes lank and greasy even a few hours after shampooing; it is caused by over-productive sebaceous glands and can also produce bad hair odour. See also pages 94–5.

The Pill
As with any other medicine that affects the hormones, contraceptive pills can be the cause of hair problems: a woman may experience excessive hair loss either while she is on the pill or when she comes off it. The pill can also cause a dry scalp and excessively oily hair.

Pityriasis
This is a loose term used for a bran-like or scaly appearance of the skin. *Pityriasis steatoides* and *pityriasis capitis* are alternative names for common dandruff. *Pityriasis amientacea* is a more virulent form of dandruff, which gathers along the hair shaft as well as over the scalp. Pityriasis should not be left untreated as hair loss will quickly follow.

Pregnancy and After-effects
Most pregnant women find their hair is healthier, shinier and more abundant during this time of increased oestrogen production; usually problems like oily hair are lessened or disappear. But from three to six months after the birth of the child the mother frequently suffers from hair loss. This hair loss is quite normal and the hair should soon recover; if the loss persists a trichologist should be consulted.

Psoriasis

This is a skin condition that manifests itself in red patches covered in silvery scales, which can also appear on the scalp. It doesn't itch but treatment so far is fairly unsuccessful – a shampoo containing tar may help.

Ringworm

This is a fungal infection of the skin; the scalp variety is known as *tinea capitis* and begins as a small papule, spreading concentrically and leaving scaly bald patches. It may have a pink centre. The sufferer should be immediately taken to a doctor, who will prescribe an antibiotic which will cure the ringworm.

Split Ends

Split ends are the result of hair abuse. Too much colouring, bleaching, perming or exposure to sun, wind and water produces damaged hair. Once hair has become split nothing can be done and the ends must be cut off and extra care taken with conditioning to restore health.

Thyroid Imbalance

Like hormonal, nutritional or any other glandular imbalance, this can cause hair loss, sudden dryness or lank hair.

Transplants

Hair transplants expertly done by cosmetic surgeons can be very successful; the technique is well-proven.

Trichotillomania

This is the name for the mania for pulling out one's hair – usually found in adolescent girls and menopausal women. See also page 101.

Unwanted Hair

Hair grows on most parts of the body – more profusely on some people than others – and causes distress if it is very dark or thick on the face, arms, legs or around the pubic area. Isolated hairs can be pulled out with tweezers. A medium growth on legs, arms or face (particularly around the upper lip) can be bleached, which will make it less obvious, or waxed away. Waxing is also the most satisfactory way of achieving a clean bikini-line. Legs and underarms can be shaved. The only permanent way of removing superfluous hair is by electrolysis, which is time-consuming, must be done by an expert and can be enormously expensive.

Zinc

Zinc Pyrithione is an ingredient in many effective anti dandruff shampoos.

Ways to Colour Your Hair

The natural colour of your hair is determined by the melanin in the hair shaft. Melanin is the name for the pigment granules in the shaft – there is sometimes a small amount present in the medulla (the innermost of the three layers that compose a strand of hair), but most is in the cortex or middle layer. The darker your hair, the darker the melanin. Your natural hair colour is decided in the womb, but much can be done to improve or alter it if you wish. If you don't like your natural colour, you can change it. You can have any colour you want, but to change the colour for good means tampering with the structure of the hair shaft, which is potentially dangerous if it is not done with infinite care. Modern techniques have made it easier, but it is still essential to have some basic understanding of the process. The outer layer of the hair shaft, or cuticle, is made of fine overlapping cells, which must be lifted in order to get colour to penetrate and reach the cortex, where the pigment granules can be altered. The only way to do this is to use a permanent form of colouring called a dye or tint. There are other, less drastic, levels of colouring, which are satisfactory and great fun, particularly for the young, who like to change their looks as often as their moods.

Colouring processes fall into three main groups: temporary, semi-permanent and permanent.

Temporary Colour
Temporary colour or water rinsing is the mildest process. The colour will only cling to the outer layer (the cuticle), contains no bleaching agent or penetrating ingredient to alter the natural

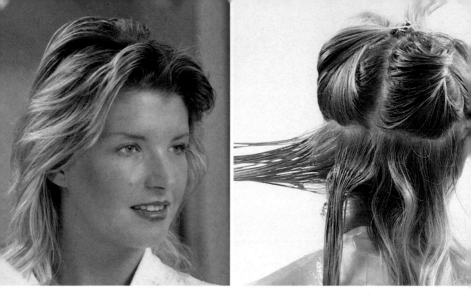

Colouring your Hair

1. ABOVE LEFT *The model's hair was a pretty blond but out of condition from the sun and years of colouring and bleaching.* **2.** ABOVE RIGHT *The hair must be coloured red to replace artificial pigment. This allows the hair to absorb the new colour. Without it the new brown would rinse away at the first wash.* **3.** *First the highlights are brushed with red pigment; they are most in need as they have been the most bleached. This is left on for thirty minutes.* **4.** *Pigment is combed through the hair.*

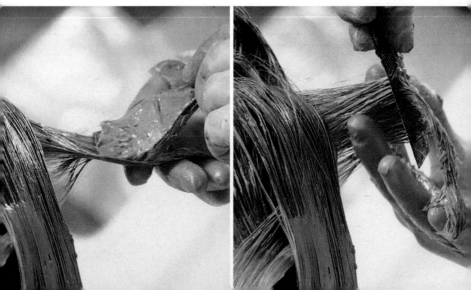

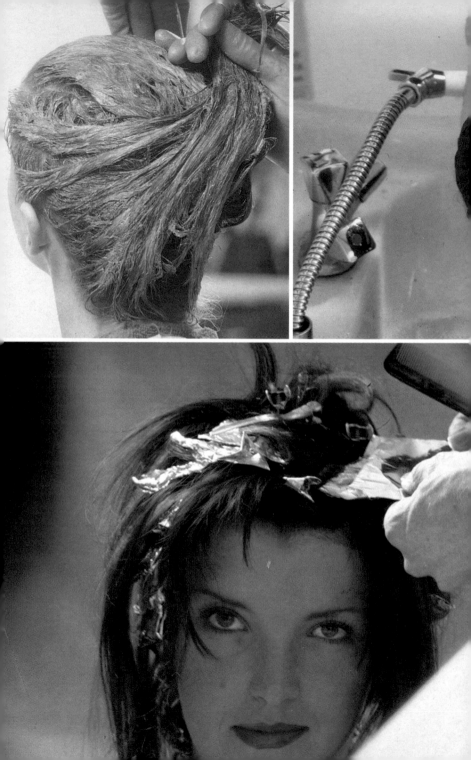

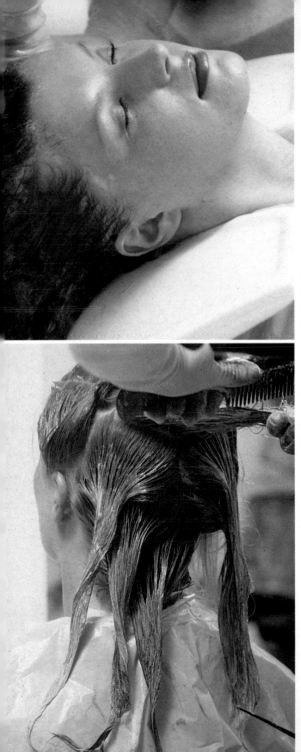

5. TOP LEFT *Colour is massaged through hair to make sure of a natural blending.*
6. TOP RIGHT *The hair is rinsed and dried.*
7. *The hair is lightened by delicately streaking with a combination of four different blonds for a natural, subtle effect. A section of the hair is taken up, and several strands are lifted from it which are then brushed with colour, wrapped in foil and left until the colour takes hold. The result is a head strewn with fine blond lights.*
8. *Conditioner is applied every time the hair is rinsed.*

Sandra Lousada

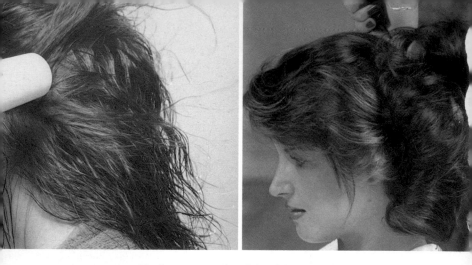

9. ABOVE LEFT *The hair is rinsed and dried for the last time.* **10.** ABOVE RIGHT *Then it is brushed into a soft knot.* **11.** BELOW *The hair is transformed by the careful treatment it has received. It has regained its glow of health.*

Sandra Lousada

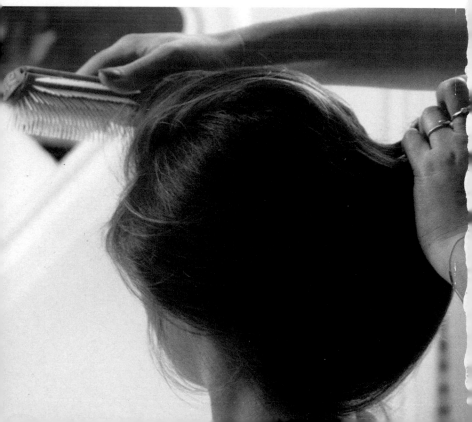

colour underneath and will disappear during the next shampoo. A colour rinse will only change the tone of the hair – shading it up or down – not the actual colour. Colour rinses are useful for improving tinted hair between applications, if the hair has faded in the sun or become brassy from bleaching – but should not be used too often for this purpose, as the coating on the cuticle may have a dulling effect over the tint. They are excellent for cleaning and brightening the tone of grey or white hair but will do nothing to cover it up.

Temporary colours are usually applied after shampooing and normally need no skin-patch test, as they are hypo-allergenic. They are simple to apply at home, but read the instructions carefully.

Semi-Permanent Colour

Semi-permanent colourants provide a medium amount of colour intensity but contain no bleaching agent so cannot alter the basic colour. They *do* contain a penetrating agent, so the depth of colour within the limits of the natural range can be altered. This depth will gradually fade away in four to six weeks, a little intensity being lost every time the hair is shampooed, until it returns to its original shade. Thus, they can enrich mouse-brown, polish a dull blond, enhance the red tones in brown hair, reduce or reveal the copper tone in red hair.

Semi-permanent colourants are useful for disguising the first grey hairs, but the effect will be more like highlighting, as there is only a certain amount of coverage; once the grey hairs become the majority, a permanent tint is the only way to cover them satisfactorily. Like temporary rinses, they usually have a built-in conditioner and are therefore useful in revitalizing dull hair – giving it added colour and lustre.

Semi-permanent colour is fairly easy to apply at home, but it is necessary to carry out a skin-patch test twenty-four hours beforehand and to follow the instructions exactly.

Permanent Colour

All permanent colourants have a toxic base and it is therefore essential to carry out a skin-patch test twenty-four hours in advance, whether you are planning to do the tint at home or to have it done by a professional colourist. It is also a good idea to do a 'strand test' at the same time. A hairdresser will normally do a skin-patch test behind your ear, but if you are colouring your hair at home, the inside of the elbow is easier to reach and observe. A small amount of tint should be mixed and applied to the skin – about a square inch is enough – and left for twenty-four hours, making sure it isn't rubbed or washed off. If there is any reaction at all, don't use the product. The strand test is done like this: cut off 30–40 strands of hair from different parts of the head, close to the scalp; using the remainder of the product used for the patch test, follow the instructions to the letter. Then study the results in strong daylight. Remember that everyone's hair colour is different, so the result is unlikely to be identical with that on the packet. What happens to those few test strands will happen to your entire head, so be sure you are happy with the colour before going ahead.

Permanent colourants – or dyes or tints, which are all more or less the same – contain both penetrating and bleaching agents (to reach through the cuticle and alter the pigment granules in the cortex) and, of course, the colour the hair is going to become (called an oxidation dye), which is mixed with the bleach. The bleach strips the granules of colour and makes the cortex porous and ready to absorb the dye and produce the change of colour. It is possible to achieve good results with permanent tints for home use, providing the colour is not to be changed too much, but, for really satisfactory effects and dramatic switches of colour, permanent tints are best applied in a salon, where the colourist can mix individual shades and time the process exactly according to the hair's texture. Fine hair absorbs colour more readily, coarse hair resists it. The only way colouring can go wrong is if it is wrongly applied. If this happens, not only will the colour be a surprise, but the hair can be badly damaged. Therefore, it is vital that permanent hair colour, whether applied at home or in a salon, is used correctly. If you are thinking of a radical alteration in your hair colour – changing from brunette or blond to red, for instance – it is a good idea to try on some wigs of the colour you have in mind. This will give you a chance to see if it really suits you and to discuss it with the colourist who is going to apply the tint. He or she will be trained in colour blending as well as application and give expert advice on the suitability of the colour you have chosen.

Bleaching on its own decolourizes the hair and gives an old-fashioned solid-white blond effect. It is much prettier on a whole head when used with several shades of tint for a more natural multi-toned effect. Bleaching is a vital part of the permanent tinting process, as it is necessary to remove the existing natural colour before imposing a new one. Done correctly, it will cause no damage to the hair, but over-bleaching makes the hair excessively dry, brittle and prone to breakage and split ends.

Streaking, highlighting and *tipping* all use a bleaching process.

Streaking involves narrow ribbons of light colour usually applied round the face, following the movement of the hair or the line of the cut. The bleach is painted on in lines down the full length of the hair, left until the desired shade is obtained, then rinsed thoroughly and either combined with a toning rinse or shampooed with the rest of the hair and conditioned.

Highlighting, sometimes called *frosting,* usually involves drawing small sections of hair through holes in a plastic cap, applying the bleach to these strands and wrapping them in tinfoil. (It can also be done without the plastic cap, just using tinfoil.) The advantage of this method is that the bleach is kept at different distances from the scalp and roots of the hair, so that as the hair grows out it blends in with the natural hair and doesn't leave an ugly regrowth line. When the desired colour is reached, the tinfoil and/or cap are removed, the bleach rinsed off and the whole head either toned with a semi-permanent toner, or shampooed and conditioned.

Tipping, sometimes called *feathering*, means that the bleach is just applied to the ends. Again the plastic cap with holes may be used, although on short hair the bleach is often painted on. This is most effective if two or three shades are chosen.

It is difficult to do any of these lightening effects successfully at home as they rely on the precise application of the bleach – faultless timing and shading-in with the rest of the hair – which is best left in the hands of the expert colourist. But with the help of a friend you may achieve a satisfactory result.

Hair should not be permanently waved for at least two weeks before or after tinting.

Natural Vegetable Dyes
Natural vegetable dyes are non-toxic and do not interfere with the structure of the hair. They cling to the cuticle or outer layer and do not penetrate the cortex or middle layer. They leave the hair shining and full of body. It usually takes several applications to achieve a colour that would be reached in one salon visit and one application of modern tint.

Henna has been used as a hair colourant for centuries and has recently become enormously popular with the revival of interest in herbal medicine, natural cosmetics and general health-consciousness. Henna dye is made from the *Lawsonia alba* plant which grows all along the North African coast and into the Middle East, from Morocco to Iran. The Moroccan henna is the lightest in colour and conditioning value, the Iranian the richest, being deeper red and full of conditioning properties and therefore the most sought after. The leaves of the plant are dried, then crushed into a powder, which is mixed with water. (Some colourists like to use black coffee or other naturally coloured liquids, and add lemon juice or vinegar to the paste.)

Henna reacts differently not only on different coloured hair, but also on the same hair under different conditions. Therefore, it is essential to make a strand test before commencing the application.

Try experimenting. It is possible to henna your hair red, rich brown with shades of red highlights or deep chestnut. The best results are obtained with hair that is naturally brunette or black, and the new colour will last several months.

For the best results go to a professional colourist, who will know what results are likely to be achieved with your hair colour as well as the source of the henna and how much orange-red pigment it contains. If you want to just brighten and condition your hair at home, try one of the temporary shampoos, which will add gloss and highlights and give you some idea of whether you want a stronger, more permanent change. As natural henna is non-toxic, it is not necessary to do a skin-patch test first and it is very useful for people with sensitive skins. Henna should never be used on hair that has been chemically tinted – it is even more difficult to control the resulting tone of the colour – and is not very satisfactory as a covering for grey hair, as it is likely to turn orange. Compound hennas are available, but these contain metallic substances and should be used according to the instructions – they should not be treated as natural vegetable dyes or be expected to work in the same way.

Camomile, when infused, has a lightening effect on hair and is most successful on blond or naturally fair hair. Depending on the strength of the infusion and the number of times it is applied, it will produce a colour from pale to bright yellow.

Marigold applied as an infusion will impart soft reddish-yellow tones to highly bleached or white hair.

Saffron – the root, not the powder used in cooking – can give a bright yellow tint to fair or blond hair but needs many applications. The dye is made by boiling the root for at least half an hour.

Sage should be infused like camomile and will dull grey hair, producing a brown tone. Mix it with strong tea for a darker colour.

Walnut will also give a brown tone to grey hair. The colourant is obtained by boiling walnuts for several hours and using the resulting liquid as a rinse, which can be stored and used when needed.

Hair and Diet

Whatever your age, if you want healthy hair, you must eat properly. Diet is the most effective way to control hair health – the good things are the natural foods, fresh fruit and vegetables, proteins, lots of water, plus extra vitamin B in the form of Brewers' Yeast tablets. The bad things are too many dairy products, animal fat, sugar, salt and spices – spices create no problem in a hot climate but in cooler places can be the cause of scalp problems.

It's up to parents to make sure that babies and children are well-nourished, but after that it's up to you – and it's not just your hair that benefits; your whole body will function better and you will feel that much fitter and more energetic. This kind of diet has nothing to do with slimming – it's a balanced way of eating for a lifetime; following it, your weight should remain stable and your hair healthy.

Work out your eating plan on a daily basis, using the following as a guide line. GOOD for you are:

Protein: lean meat for vitamin E, and liver (once a week) for vitamin B: fish for iron and vitamin A; eggs (but one a day is enough) for vitamin B and vitamin D, which is also found in liver and tuna fish.
Fresh vegetables: particularly green ones like spinach and broccoli for vitamin C; carrots for vitamin A. (Make it a rule to cook vegetables lightly to keep all the goodness intact.)
Salad: all the greens and raw vegetables such as lettuce, tomatoes and endive for vitamin A; watercress, mustard, spinach and

cauliflower for vitamin K; celery, radishes, carrots and avocados for iron. (You can make a delicious meal from a bowl of salad – add a few nuts for vitamin E and currants for more iron.)

Fresh fruit: lots of it and whatever is in season.

Roughage: wholewheat cereal, or bran or wholemeal bread (use polyunsaturated margarine rather than butter) for vitamin B; brown rice for vitamins E and B; baked potatoes for vitamin C inside and iron in the skin.

Liquid: lots of water, at least six glasses a day.

Sweetening: honey when possible.

AVOID, or cut out if you can, the following:

Milk and milk products like ice-cream, cream, sour cream, cheese.

Sugary items like cakes, biscuits, puddings, chocolates, sweets.

Salty items like potato crisps, pickles, sauces.

Over-processed foods like white bread, white sugar, white rice.

Fried foods (grilled, poached and baked are better).

Caffeine drinks (coffee, tea, colas).

Alcoholic drinks.

Cigarettes.

A nutritious, balanced diet should provide you with all the vitamins you need, but if you feel run-down, have been on antibiotics or for some reason your hair looks lack-lustre, take supplements of iron and vitamins B, C, K and E. Vitamins A and D should *not* be taken in supplementary pill form.

Recipes for Healthy Hair

Orange and Tomato Soup

2 lb (0.9 kg) ripe tomatoes
1 medium onion
1 medium carrot
1 bay leaf
8 peppercorns
1 small piece lemon rind
pinch salt
2 pints (1.1 ℓ) stock

½ oz (15 g) margarine
1 oz (30 g) plain flour
juice and rind of ½ orange
1 small teaspoon sugar
1 carton natural unsweetened
  yogurt
fresh basil

Skin and remove pips from tomatoes. Place them with the peeled, sliced onion and carrot, bay leaf, peppercorns, lemon rind, salt and stock in a saucepan. Cover and bring to the boil, then simmer for half an hour. Put in the blender to liquidize, then return to the pan, adding margarine and flour; bring back to the boil and boil for 2–3 minutes (until thick), whisking continuously. Stir in grated orange rind, juice, sugar. Remove from heat and when cool stir in the yogurt. Garnish with chopped fresh basil. (Serves 6–8)

Tomato Jelly

2 tablespoons gelatine
1 pint (0.6 ℓ) tomato juice
2 lemons

1¼ pints (0.7 ℓ) chicken stock
salt and pepper
Worcestershire sauce

Sprinkle gelatine on tomato juice in a heavy saucepan. Add grated rind of 1 lemon and the chicken stock. Bring slowly to the boil, stirring continuously; when boiling, lower the heat and cook for a further five minutes. Strain through a fine sieve and add pepper, salt, lemon juice and a dash of Worcestershire sauce. Put into a mould or individual cocotte dishes and set in refrigerator for 2–3 hours. Serve with chopped chives or a sauce of natural unsweetened yogurt seasoned with lemon juice, salt, pepper and cayenne. (Serves 6–8)

Cold Cucumber and Dill Soup

4 peeled cucumbers	2 pints (0.6 ℓ) chicken stock
2 tablespoons chopped fresh dill	large carton natural yogurt
salt and pepper	

Make a purée of the cucumbers and pour into a large bowl. Add dill, salt, pepper and chicken stock. Stir well, then chill for several hours. Just before serving, add enough yogurt to get the desired consistency. Sprinkle a little extra dill on top. (Serves 6–8)

Crudités with Garlic Dip

Arrange a selection of fresh raw vegetables in a basket or bowl and place a small bowl of dip in the centre. A good mixture is cauliflower, fennel, radishes, carrots, celery and small tomatoes. For the dip, season a carton of natural unsweetened yogurt with salt and freshly ground black pepper and add a crushed clove of garlic.

Simple Starters

Serve ripe melons with a quarter of lemon instead of sugar.
Sprinkle avocado pears with salt and pepper and a squeeze of lemon juice.
Grill half a grapefruit with a tiny amount of thin honey.
Grate some carrots and dress them with orange juice, chopped mint, salt and pepper.

Green Bean and Prawn Salad

Combine cold cooked thin French beans with cold cooked artichoke hearts and place in a bowl. Surround with segments of fresh grapefruit and cover with prawns and a sprinkling of lumpfish roe. Season with salt, freshly ground black pepper and lemon juice. This makes an excellent lunch dish.

Risotto

12 oz (340 g) brown rice	4 oz (115 g) chopped tomatoes
1½ pints (0.9 ℓ) chicken stock	4 oz (115 g) grated parmesan
salt	cheese
5 oz (140 g) chopped onions	chopped fresh basil
4 oz (115 g) margarine	

Put rice in a pan with stock and a pinch of salt. Bring to the boil, cover tightly and simmer for 45 minutes. Meanwhile, cook the onion in the margarine until just turning brown and add the tomatoes just before combining with the cooked rice. Serve with grated cheese, a little chopped fresh basil, if it is in season, and a green salad. (Serves 6–8)

Grilled Chicken with Lemon
Rub a little oil over chicken pieces on both sides. Sprinkle with salt, pepper, rosemary and a good squeeze of lemon juice and grill well until cooked through, or bake slowly in the oven. Serve with small baked potatoes and lightly cooked courgettes.

Kedgeree

2–4 oz (55–115 g) margarine	4 cups cold boiled brown rice
16 oz (455 g) cooked flaked	salt and pepper
fish (one with a good	pinch of nutmeg
flavour – salmon or smoked	4 hard-boiled eggs
haddock, for instance)	1 lemon

Melt the margarine and stir in the fish and rice. Season with salt, pepper and nutmeg and add chopped egg whites. Heat very gently until hot right through, then pile in a dish. Rub the egg yolks through a sieve and sprinkle over the top. Serve with lemon sections and a green salad. (Serves 6–8)

Baked Bananas
Peel and put in shallow oven-proof dish, pour over a little thin honey and lots of lemon juice and bake slowly.

Melon and Plum Salad

1 melon	10 oz (285 g) orange juice
1½ lb (0.7 kg) plums	2 oz (55 g) honey

Remove seeds from the melon, peel and cut the flesh into cubes. Wash, stone and cut the plums in segments. Mix the fruit and add the orange juice, in which the honey has been dissolved. Chill.

Baked Apples
Core the apples and put in a shallow oven-proof dish. Stuff the centres with honey, raisins, dates, cloves, cinnamon, marmalade. Sprinkle with a little brown sugar and add about a quarter of an inch of water. Bake in a moderate oven, basting occasionally, for about 45 minutes. Serve hot or cold.

Raspberry Ginger Cream

12 oz (340 g) fresh or frozen raspberries	ground ginger to taste
2 tablespoons thin honey	½ pint (0.3 ℓ) natural unsweetened yogurt

Thaw berries if frozen, drain thoroughly and separate. Mix honey, ginger and yogurt and fold in the raspberries gently. Chill for at least an hour. Before serving, stir again gently to blend in any juice.

Hair and Exercise   A healthy body means healthy hair. Any routine of exercises will include some to rev up the circulation – this will benefit the hair most, bringing oxygen through the bloodstream to feed the hair follicles. Five or ten minutes a day will help, though a longer session is recommended. Exercises also relax the mind and body muscles and ease tension – all of which mean a general lessening of stress, one of hair's worst enemies.

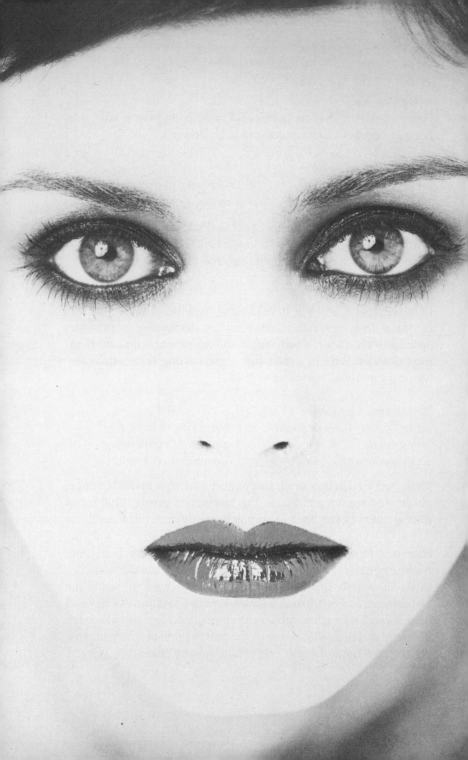

Make-up

When you are about to make up your face, take a long hard look at yourself in the mirror. Make-up can be natural or dramatic, light or heavy, can enhance your natural features or act as a mask or disguise. So, before you begin, you must decide which effect you are after. However extreme you want the finished look to be, the trick is to use a light hand – always start gently and build up the colour, shade and shape. It's much easier to add than take away, and less time-consuming – at least until you've become adept at handling the pencils, palettes, powders, creams and brushes that are part of the modern cosmetic kit.

For a dramatic effect like that in the picture, you must use a foundation that gives good coverage in order to blank out your personality – probably much heavier than normal and possibly a much lighter or darker shade than you usually wear – before starting to bring back your features, shading and shaping where needed, and adding colour. You will need lots of loose translucent powder to set this foundation – dust it on lavishly and brush away the excess. Then start to work on your eyes, first drawing the outline of the final shape you want with a pencil and then softening it by blending into the surrounding area, filling in with powder or cream colour, adding highlight and mascara at the end and curling the lashes. Lips must be outlined with a pencil, filled in with colour and then blotted – for a longer-lasting effect, another dusting of powder at this stage will help; then apply another coat of colour or gloss.

Now, stand away from the mirror and judge your handwork from a distance.

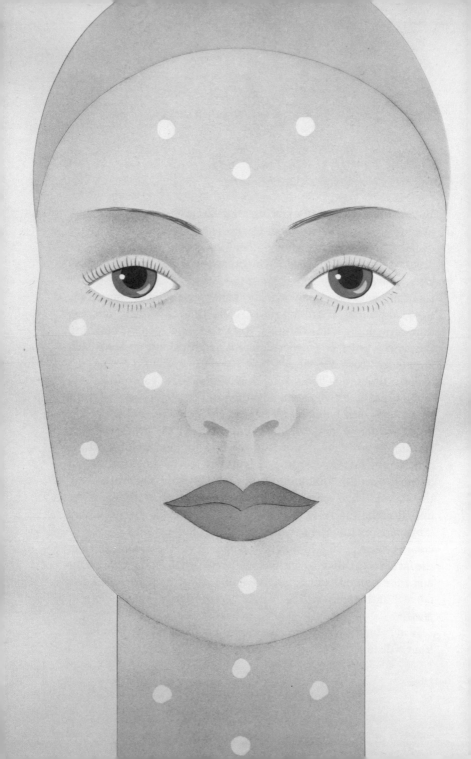

Make-up Routine

Stage One: Cleanse, Tone, Moisturize
Before starting to apply your make-up, you must give yourself the best possible base to work on. This means skin in good condition – which comes from the correct, regular skin-care regime for your skin type, a well-balanced diet (including lots of mineral water), enough sleep, and enough exercise to rev up your circulation. All these ingredients contribute to the appearance of your skin – its clarity, tone and texture. Every time you start to make up, check first that your skin is scrupulously clean. What you cleanse with depends on your skin type and your personal preference for a lotion, cream, foam or soap-and-water. Having cleansed, wipe away any last traces of dirt, debris or grease with a skin freshener or toner – again, which you use depends on your skin type: non-alcoholic fresheners are for dry and sensitive skins, those with alcohol (usually called astringents) are only for oily skins. People with combination skins (patches of dry skin or a t-shape of greasiness down the centre of the face) are wise to use both, or a toner with only a tiny amount of alcohol, diluted (by soaking a cotton-wool pad in water first) for the dry patches.

Cleanse and Tone
Use cool water or non-alcoholic skin tonic.

Moisturize
Dot all over face and neck and blend gently. Don't use too much. Excess moisturizer will only evaporate on the skin and make it drier.

The last step in preparation is moisturizing. Moisturizers are probably the biggest breakthrough in skin care in recent years – they provide a film over the skin that prevents its natural moisture from escaping and causing dehydration, which is the main cause of wrinkles and skin ageing. They also protect the skin from environmental damage – from wind, cold, sun (providing they contain a sunscreen), pollution – especially when no foundation is worn, and help enormously in the smooth application of foundation, as they leave the skin in a soft, supple condition.

Tinted moisturizers are very helpful under foundation to help balance out skin tones. A green tint will tone down redness; mauve reduces sallowness; apricot will warm up a washed-out pallor. But, don't use too much or the result will veer towards the opposite extreme.

Stage Two: Foundation and Camouflage
Foundation, or base, should be considered as a skin improver, something that will give the impression of better, smooth and even-

Dark Circles under the Eyes
Find the dark patches by lowering your head and looking up into a mirror. Gently dot concealer sparingly on the circle and blend by patting with the fingertip. Don't rub or drag. If circle is accompanied by a 'bag' don't let the concealer go over it – this only accentuates it. Powder very lightly if necessary – but avoid powdering under the eyes if possible as it sinks in and deepens tiny lines.

Foundation
Choose to match your skin tone. Apply with damp sponge or fingers. Be careful to blend around nose and chin and fade away under chin. Don't take it into hair line, nor heavily under eyes – it can make tiny lines look deeper than they are.

Eric Boman

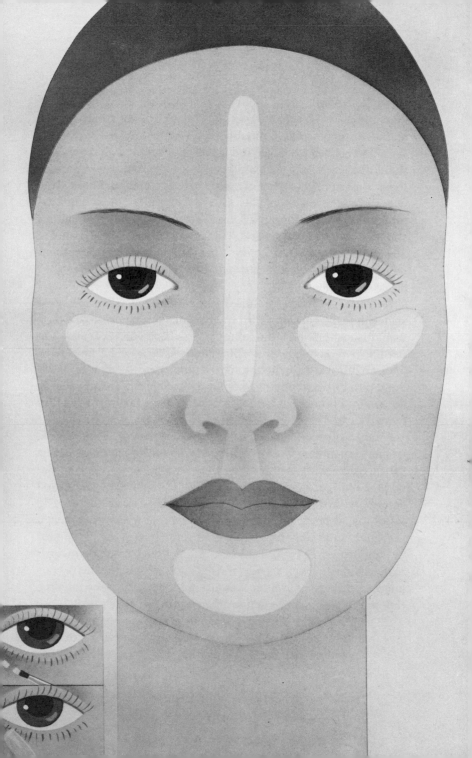

toned skin, while the product itself is almost invisible. Heavy foundation is old-fashioned and ageing; it should never appear mask-like or obvious. Contemporary foundations are light and should be applied sparingly and blended in well. The shade chosen should be as close to your natural skin tone as possible, so that there is no sudden change of colour between chin and neck. This way the end result should be an all-over quality of tone and texture, with just a transparent glaze. Never select your foundation shade by trying it on the back of the hand – the skin here is almost always a totally different colour from that on your face. Test them on the side of your cheek, just above the jawbone, and make your decision in a good light.

Only the very young, or those lucky enough to have near-perfect skin, can really get away with wearing no foundation at all if they want to look their best. But, many people have good skin and only need help in certain areas – chin, forehead or nose, for instance – and can just use the foundation to improve tone in patches, blending it into the surrounding skin for an even effect. In summer, or for sports, a bronze gel is often sufficient, providing just a healthy overall glow.

Foundations are available in various forms – liquids, gels, creams, cream-foams, or solid creams in sticks, blocks or cakes. Which you choose is a matter of how much clarity or cover you want – and personal preference. Most of them are water-in-oil emulsions, with some oil-free liquid formulas especially for oily skins; the all-in-one mixtures of cream and powder which give a very matt finish are best for oily skins too. They should be applied by dotting over the central area of the face, then blending outwards with a damp (not wet) sponge and finishing off with the tips of your fingers; pay particular attention around the hairline and jaw-line that there is no sudden change of tone – and around nostrils, nose and lips. A bit of camouflage is often necessary to cover up the odd spot, patch of discolouration under eyes, scar or other blemish. A heavy cream foundation is suitable, in the same tone as your normal one but in a much lighter shade; also, there are special concealers in sticks or thick cream formulas available, sometimes with their own sponge applicators, which are easy to use. Dot the concealer on the required area, then pat or lightly press it in – use a small amount to start with; you can always add more – then blend the outer edges carefully into the surrounding skin. The technique for covering blemishes is the same whether you are wearing foundation or just moisturizer.

Stage Three: Shape, Blush, Powder

Blusher has taken over the role of old-fashioned rouge. Before there was rouge, or before it was considered permissible to wear it, women used to pinch their cheeks to bring up the colour, knowing it was the best natural way of making the most of their looks. Now, blusher is probably the single most flattering piece of make-up you can possess. It comes in cream, gel or powder form and is the next step in your make-up routine if you choose the cream variety, which includes pencils; if you choose powder blusher, it should be applied after face powder; if you choose the gel variety it is applied over foundation, and face powder shouldn't be used at all – it is designed for the most transparent effect and so would serve no purpose.

Whichever variety you choose, how it is placed on the cheek is vital. The trick is to stare straight ahead of you into a mirror and put a finger directly below your eyeball on your cheekbone. The blusher should be placed there and then blended along the cheekbone towards the hairline. Be careful not to take it too close to your nose, eye or the hollow of your cheek. It's meant to make you look healthy, not feverish. Nobody's face is perfect and bad contouring or shaping can easily end up looking like dirty marks or a heavy bruise. So, if you want to hollow your cheeks, slim your nose or reduce your jaw-line, use the minimum of colour and the lightest touch. Choose a darker shade of foundation or blusher, avoid red tones and test the effects on a friend – to make sure you haven't

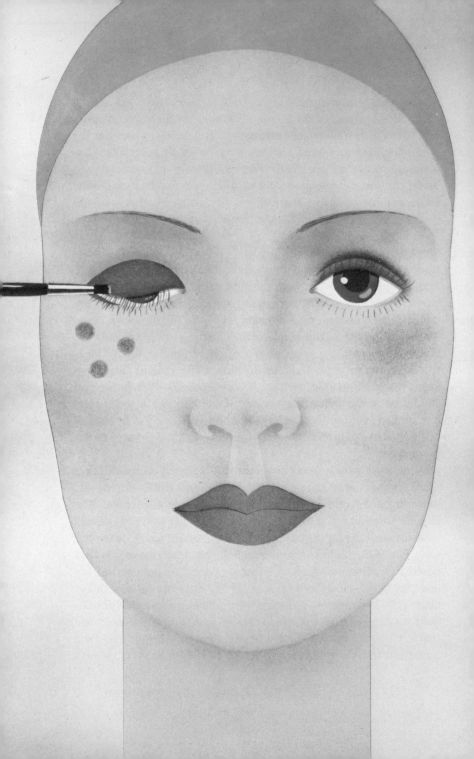

made matters worse. It's often better to play up your good points and forget what you consider the bad ones – they're never so obvious to other people.

As far as blusher colour is concerned, either pinch your cheeks and choose the shade nearest this natural blush or pick one similar in colour to the clothes you wear next to your face. For instance, with wine, crimson or purple clothes, try deep to medium true pink; with orangey shades, peach or tawny tones work best; and with beiges or tans, try the tawny corals or russets. Anything that is pearlized or has gold or silver in it should be left for evening make-up – and they are particularly effective with a tan.

If you want your make-up to last through the day or evening without requiring much repair, face powder is an essential part of the routine. Keep loose powder on your dressing table and carry a compact of pressed powder around with you. Translucent powders are the most popular now – used not to add any colour but to set make-up. They should be used after any cream product you are applying (blusher or cream eye colour; if used after the first coat of lipstick has been applied and blotted, they help stop 'bleeding'

Cream Eye Shadow

Apply after the foundation, before the powder. Use a brush and blend with a clean brush or fingertips, all over lid or wherever it suits you. Fade away at the edges and put a little under the eye if you like, use translucent powder when you powder your face.

Cream Blusher

Put on the cheek bone. Find the correct place by squeezing your index finger on the outer edge of the bone under your eye, your thumb beneath; it should make an 'egg' shape, the wide bit nearer to the outside edges of the face. Blend well, not too far in towards the nose. Left half of the face shows the action, right half the effect.

around the lips) but before any powder colour. A good trick is to dust over much more powder than necessary and then brush off the excess – this ensures its lasting effect. Check that there are no dusty patches and that it is well blended around the nostrils and below the lips.

Stage Four: Eyes

Your eyes are one of your most unique features, and they're one of the most sensitive too. They instantly reflect emotions, respond to wind, dust, glare, lack of sleep, a smoky atmosphere, alcohol and over-indulgence, ill-health and even your sleeping position. It's a good idea to protect them from wind, dust and glare with sunglasses, to keep the delicate skin around the eye area well moisturized with a special eye cream, to remove eye make-up with special eye make-up remover, and to try not to get into the habit of sleeping with your eyes scrunched into the pillow, as this can encourage lines. A healthy diet, lots of mineral water, plenty of sleep and exercise all help to keep your eyes bright and sparkling.

Treating your eyes with care is an investment and ensures they look their best. Furthermore, the eye area provides infinite scope

Powder Blusher

Apply this the same way as cream blusher but with a brush after powdering your face. Right side of face shows the action, left side the effect.

Powder Eye Shadow

After powdering the face apply eye shadow with applicator or brush, all over lids, in the socket, on the browbone, under lower lid, wherever it suits you best. Apply lightly, blend carefully at the edges – make sure it goes all the way into your lashes. Be sparing, powder shadows can make the skin look crepey if too heavily applied.

Eric Boman

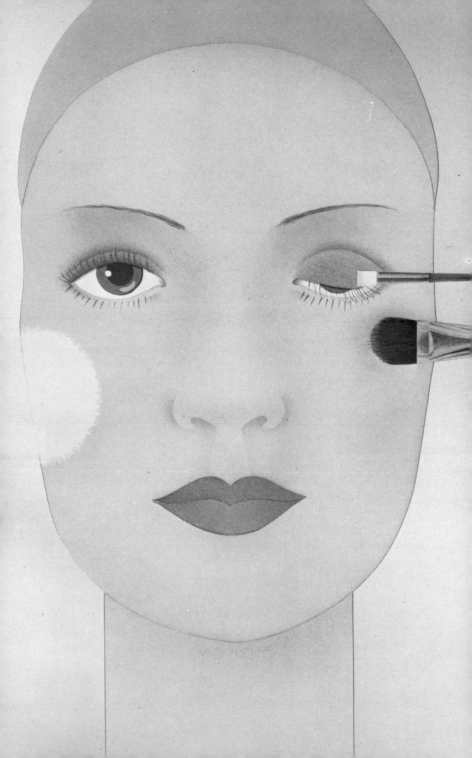

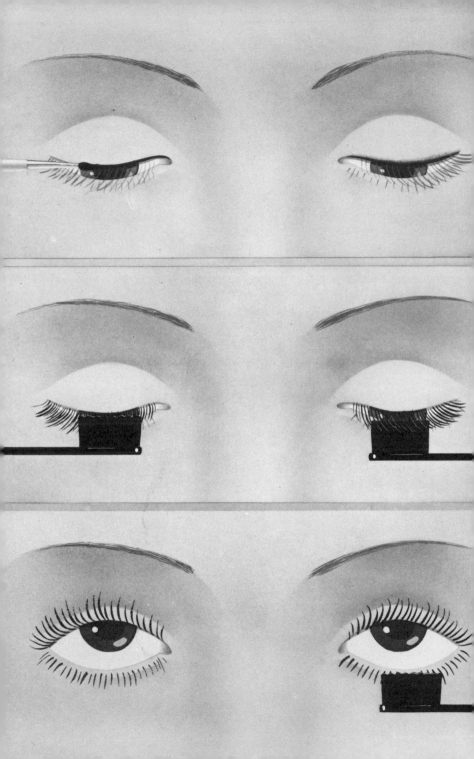

for the most imaginative make-up. It can be just a question of enhancing the eyes naturally with neutral shadows and mascara or really going to town with colour and shape. Whichever it is to be, your eyes are where contact is normally made with another person, the feature they see first; it is important to know how to use make-up so they always look good.

First decide whether you are going for an unmade-up look or a dramatic effect – then choose your colours and products accordingly.

From the vast array available, choose the products you find easiest to use. Successful eye make-up relies on skilful application and it is much better not to be too adventurous at first until you are sure of the effect and have had enough time to practise.

Eye colours come in liquid, gel, powder or cream form; in bottles, tubes, pots, compacts, sticks or pencils. Pencils have made life a great deal easier for the average person as they are easy to control for shape and, being a cream formula, blend in well. A set of make-up brushes, sponges and combs will also be useful, keeping edges neat, eyelashes in place and applying products that don't come with their own applicator. It is essential to keep everything very clean, to avoid any possible irritation to the eyes.

Start with your chosen product on the lid, near the lashes and in the socket – draw the lines according to the shape of your eyes. How much lid shows, how much space you have between socket and brow, whether they are wide, deep- or close-set, all have a

Eyeliner

Draw with a pointed brush from inner to outer corner of upper lid. Make sure to apply it right into lash base. Don't flick it up at the end, just take a damp brush and soften the whole line by smudging the edge very gently (cake liners are best for this).

bearing on the placing of shadow – see pages 62–5 for how to overcome problems and make the best of your natural shape.

Next, use an eyeliner close to the lashes, or kohl pencil on the inner rims, if you are going to. This needs a steady hand or will look very messy. This is also the moment to use eyelash curlers, which, once you've mastered the instrument, are very useful – they make mascara application easier, open up the eyes and can create the illusion of longer, thicker lashes. It is very important not to pull eyelash curlers away from the lashes before fully opening the instrument! Then highlight over the bone below the eyebrow – transparent skin tones are best for day in cream, pink or beige shades; keep high shine or metallic gleam for evening – and add a touch on the cheekbone below the outer corner of the eye.

If you have very sparse or short eyelashes you may like to add false ones. Whole strips are inclined to look very false, but a few single ones added to your own, particularly towards the outer corners, add thickness, length and can be very effective. Follow the directions exactly and, if you do use a strip, make sure it is well attached and isn't going to start lifting up at the corners.

The last step is mascara – easiest to apply is the wand, but it comes in cream or cake form too. Cream needs a good brush, as it is messy to use; the cake form usually comes with its own brush, is applied with water in several coats and is very efficient: it stays on well and the lashes don't clog. The technique for applying mascara is the same: first the top side of the upper lashes, stroking the colour down, then the underside of the top lashes, stroking the colour up, and lastly the lower lashes. Be careful there are no blobs of mascara left on the lashes and that they are well separated – a combined lash brush and comb is good – any colour that has touched the surrounding skin can be removed with a cotton bud. The best effect will be achieved with several light coats of mascara – this takes time but is well worth it.

Finally, look straight ahead into the mirror to check the shape you've made around your eyes; look closer to make sure everything is tidy – especially the inner corners of the eyes – and remove unwanted smudges of colour or flecks of powder with a cotton bud or sponge-stick applicator. Add a little depth to the colour in the socket if necessary – it may have soaked in a bit by this time. Brush eyebrows well to remove any trace of powder, up first, then across in the direction they grow. Then define with an eyebrow pencil if necessary – use soft, light feathery strokes and extend slightly at the ends. Lastly, brush again to blend in the pencil work. Eyebrows are an essential part of your facial character and provide a natural balance.

Fifth and Last Stage: Lips and Nails

After eyes, lips come close to being your most expressive feature. They are very mobile and sensual and your make-up must add to these qualities and never make them look stiff or dry. Fashion swings like a pendulum from lipsticks that are very dark through vivid bright colours to those that are closest to natural lip shades – and occasionally, as in the early sixties, to chalky pinks that are unnaturally pale and not very flattering, as they make the mouth look dry, but do draw attention to the eyes. One of the quickest ways to give yourself a new look is to reverse the focus you've been giving your face – for instance, if you've been wearing dark lipstick and not much eye make-up, try the opposite. This also gives you a chance to learn new make-up techniques, experiment with new products and avoid slipping into a make-up rut. Lip colours come in the conventional stick form, in tubes, compacts, pots or pencils; they range from opaque matt colours through shiny iridescent or pearlized shades to thin transparent tinted or colourless gloss. Again, pencils have made a terrific difference in helping people make up their lips successfully, but even better is to learn to use a lip brush. This way you get the cleanest possible outline – with colour filled in exactly where you want it and it should be – and, with practice you can learn the tricks that change the shape or emphasis of your mouth.

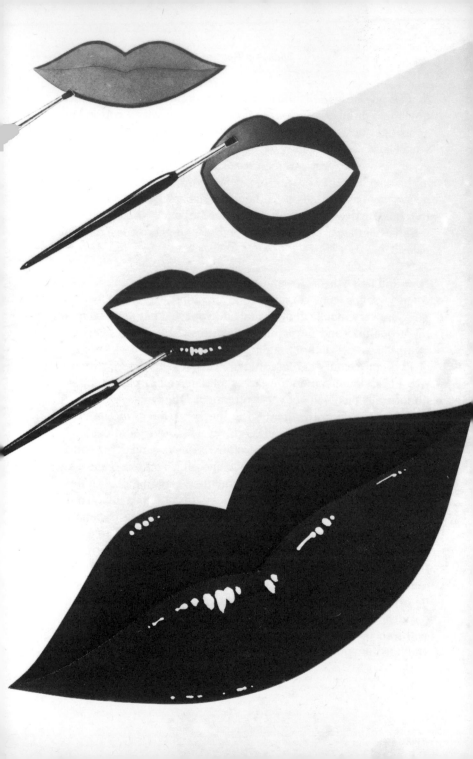

It's a good idea to have a small wardrobe of lip colours in products you find easy to use and a selection of clean brushes. When buying new colours, remember they will change when applied over your lips – a sensible place to test them is on the pad of a finger, which already has a pink tone.

When you start to make up your mouth, the outline of the lips should be rather obscure as your foundation and powder should have been blended over the edges. Outline first with a sharp pencil or lip brush in a colour that is a tone darker than the shade you're going to fill in with – you need a steady hand, so it's a good idea to rest your elbow on something solid. Then fill in with lip colour, either direct from the stick or using a lip brush. Blot, and apply another coat or add gloss – again with a lip brush; don't take the gloss right to the edges as it may cause the lipstick to run and ruin your clean outline.

Now stand away and look at yourself in a full-length mirror and check the balance of your make-up with your hair and clothes. This is particularly important for the shape of your mouth.

Don't forget how often your hands are seen in conjunction with your face – just because you've finished using them to apply your make-up doesn't mean you can dismiss them. Think how often you rest your chin on your hands, brush away a strand of hair or use your hands when you are talking. They are frequently closer to your face than you may realize.

Lipstick
Use a lip brush to put it on; powder around your mouth first (it minimizes 'bleeding'). Draw carefully and fill in with the brush or stick. Use lots of gloss. Steady your hand by resting your curled fingers on your chin. Don't make a hard different coloured line around your lips with a pencil or dark lipstick – it looks peculiar when the middle bit wears away.

You may not like nail colour, in which case nails should be buffed to a shine with special cream and a chamois leather nail buffer and the tips kept scrupulously clean and perhaps brightened underneath with a white nail pencil. If you do like nail colour, it needn't match your lip colour but should look pretty beside it whether toning or contrasting – and often the prettiest and most flattering to the hands of all are the beige or pale pink shades.

Nail polish, varnish or enamel come in bottles with their own applicator brushes and many companies offer colours that match or tone well with lipstick shades. Applying several thin coats, drying well in between and building up the colour is the best method and will prevent them chipping too soon.

However you choose to present your nails, they must be well manicured and cared for – bitten, broken or splitting nails, dry, frayed cuticles and hangnails and rough dry hands will ruin the effect of the most beautifully made-up face, hair and clothes. Hands are often a give-away on age, so to start treating them well early is an obvious investment in the future. The length and shape of nails varies with fashion and is also a question of life-style – someone who plays the piano, types or uses their hands a lot obviously cannot have long nails. Settle for nails that are all one length, healthy and well cared for – if they must be short, buff them or use a clear polish; if they are medium length, choose a colour that doesn't draw too much attention to them; don't make the mistake of ever growing them too long – talons are not attractive.

Highlighters
Apply after you have finished your make-up. Put them on with a brush and blend with your fingertips and anywhere you like, to make the skin look lively. Blend carefully so it doesn't 'sit' on the surface of the skin. Left side of face shows the action, right side, the effect.

Eric Boman

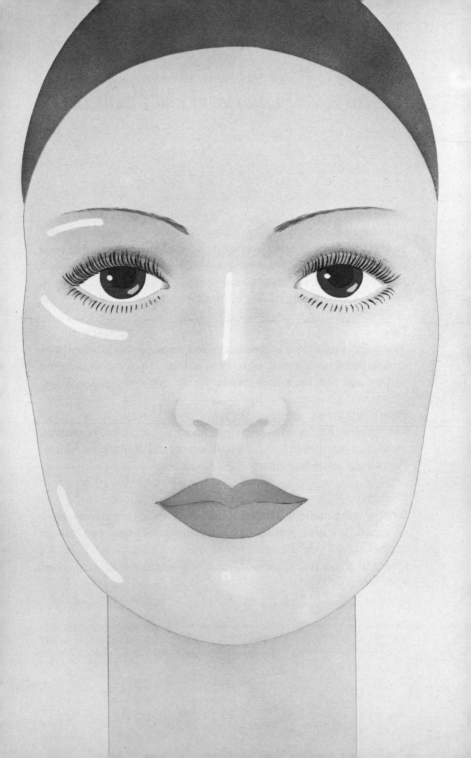

An A-Z of Equipment and Products

Applicators
Brushes that come with lip gloss, compacts of lipstick, powder blushers, powder eyeshadow; sponge-tipped sticks that come with powder or cream eyeshadows; spiral brushes that come with wand types of mascara; or tiny spatulas provided with foundation are all applicators. Your fingers are natural applicators.

Base
Also called foundation and sometimes 'make-up', this is tinted solid cream, liquid or gel designed to even out the skin tone, smooth the surface and provide a background for lip, eye and cheek colours.

Bleaching Cream
This lightens hair and is very useful for small patches of unwanted facial hair around lips etc.; if hair is very thick, dark or coarse, electrolysis is the best answer.

Blusher
Blusher is the modern term for rouge; it comes in cream form, stick or pencil, gel and powder. The creams, sticks and pencils are applied before powder; gel is best used without powder, as it's meant to give a transparent shine; the powder form is brushed on after face powder.

Three make-up stories on the following pages show step-by-step beauty including the skills of a make-up artist for the professional look, a fresh face for daytime and a make-up with shine and light for evening.

Eric Boman

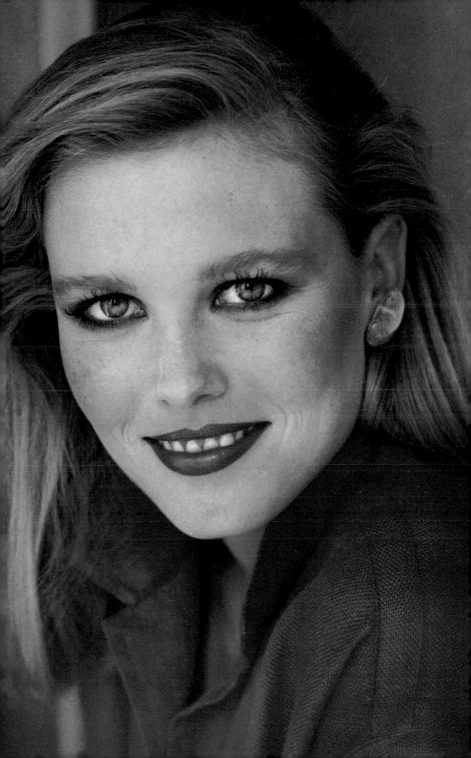

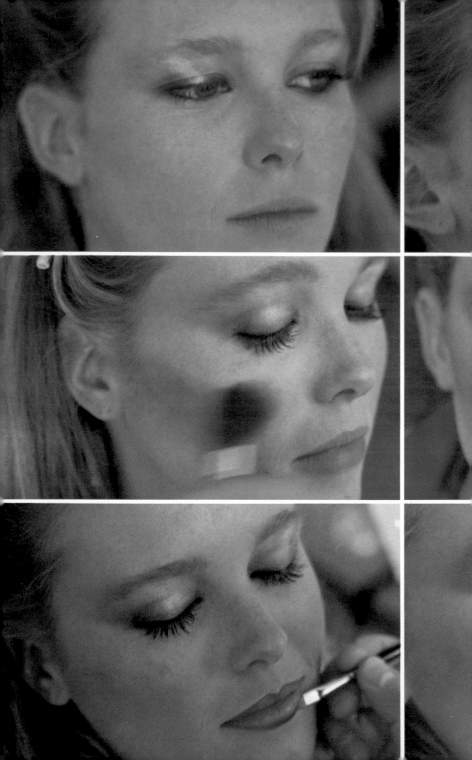

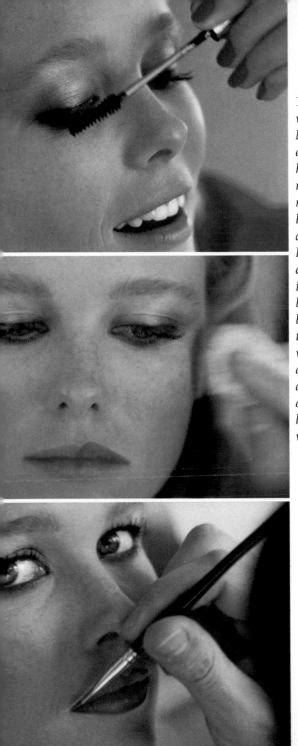

1. The face is covered with foundation and loose powder and the eyes are shaded and highlighted. 2. The model applies her own mascara, first brushing top lashes down and up, then lower lashes. 3. A dark shade of blusher is smoothed on with a brush. 4, 5 The blusher is blended to the desired strength with a small sponge and then the lipstick is applied. 6. The lips are carefully outlined before being filled in with a brush.

Eric Boman

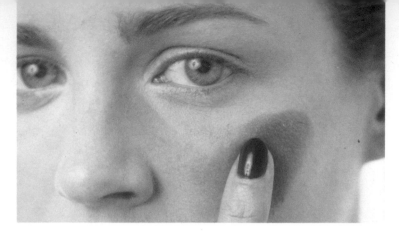

Step-by-step beauty for daytime make-up

First, smooth on a foundation neither too pale nor too tanned. Add blusher, then colour eyelids, dust over brow bones, softly rim lower lids with sponge applicator. Finish with mascara. Add shine to lips with lipgloss, over lipstick.

John Bishop

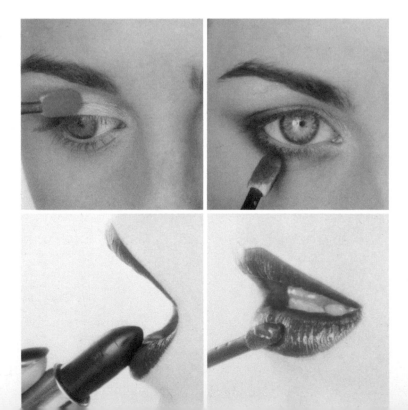

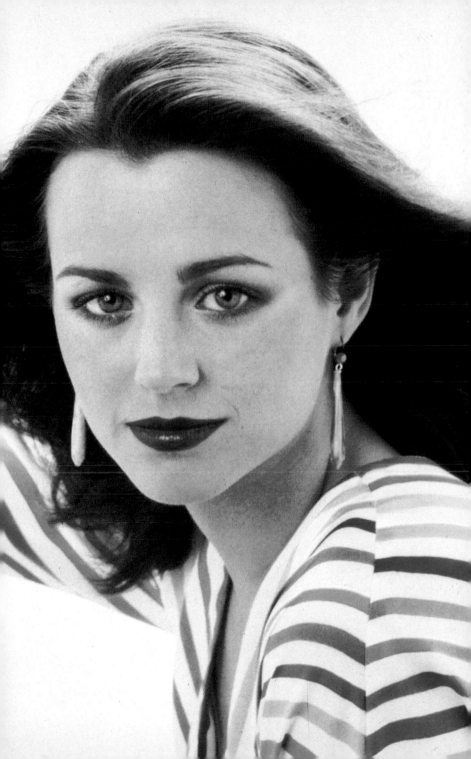

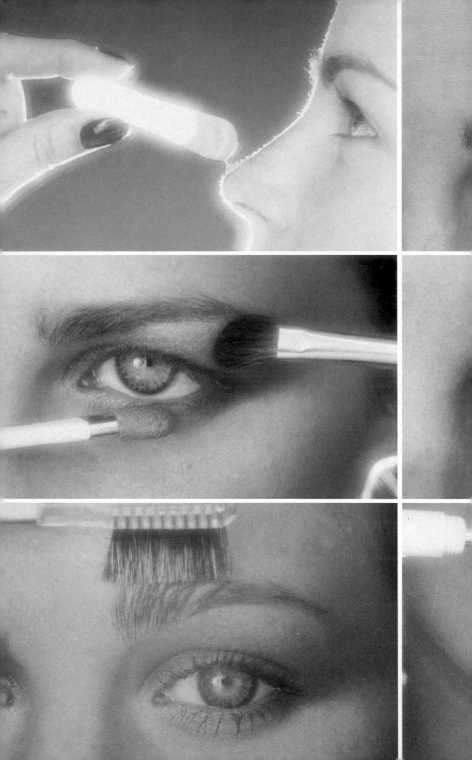

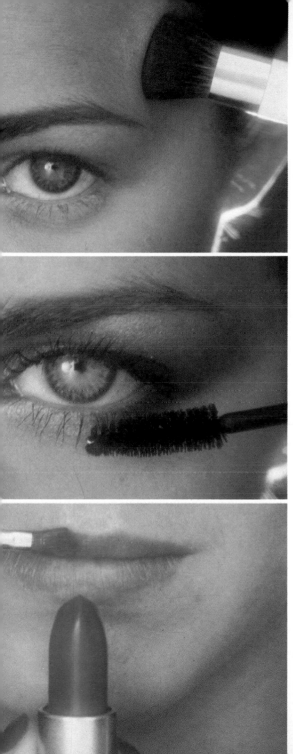

Step-by-step beauty for evening make-up
1. Cleanse skin of all trace of day make-up and apply foundation by dotting over face. 2. Blend with small light strokes. 3 & 4. With a new set of brushes apply soft clear colouring for eyes, outlining them and shading upper lids. 5. Tidy brows with eyebrow brush and comb. Apply final light touches with tulip pink blusher and translucent powder. 6. Paint lips, colour cheeks and complete make-up with a light dusting of powder.

John Bishop

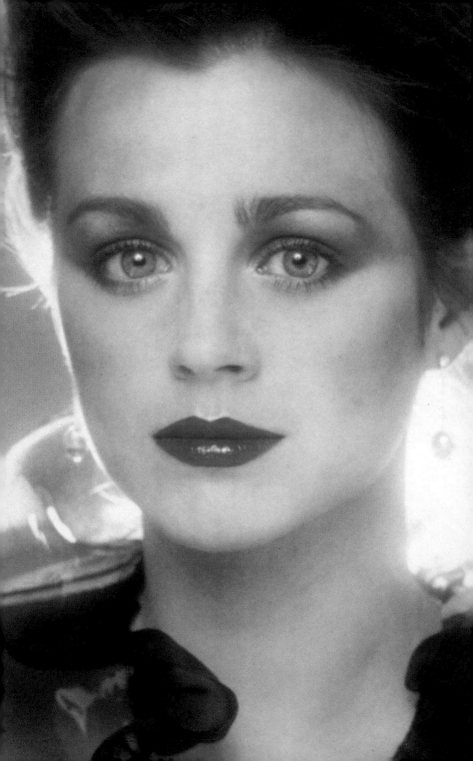

Brushes
Two or three brushes in different sizes, once you've mastered the art of using them, will help you give a professional touch to your make-up. They give cleaner lines, blend colours better. Paint-brushes from an art shop are fine; you can also buy sets of cosmetic brushes, usually with some sponge and comb applicators as well.

Buffer
An oblong pad covered in chamois leather, a buffer is used with a buffing cream to bring a natural sheen to nails without the use of enamel.

Calamine Lotion
This is a tinted medicated liquid, very useful for soothing sunburn or itchy rashes or drying spots.

Combs
Tiny plastic combs are useful for separating eyelashes and smoothing eyebrows into line.

Concealer
This is an essential part of make-up. In stick or pencil or cream form, concealers come in various shades and are designed to cover discolouration or blemishes of any kind.

Cotton Buds
These are ideal for whisking away odd specks of coloured powder or mascara and generally tidying up make-up.

Cuticle Cream
This is a nourishing cream massaged into the cuticles and bases of the nail, to feed the nail where it grows and to keep the cuticles soft and separate from the nail.

Emery Boards
These are long spatulas covered in sand paper – medium-grained on one side, fine on the other – for filing finger- and toenails.

Eyelash Curlers
These are a scissors-like device for curling short or thin lashes. They should be used before mascara. A bit of practice is required: give just a gentle squeeze, which is enough to lift the lashes; be sure and open the scissors before taking the curlers off the lashes or you will pull them out; and don't re-curl after applying mascara – the mascara will stick to the curlers and pull out the lashes.

Eye Make-up
Any colour that you apply around your eyes counts as eye make-up: eyeshadows which come in cream, stick, liquid, gel or powder form; pencils, including kohl formulas for lining the rims; eyeliner; eyebrow pencils; mascara.

Eye Make-up Remover
This is a cleaner specifically designed to remove eye make-up efficiently. The eye and surrounding area are very sensitive and it is important that all make-up is thoroughly removed.

Fading Cream
This is a product designed to fade freckles and brown spots.

False Eyelashes
These can be bought in pairs (in various lengths and colours) or in long strips, from which you can take just one or two lashes and apply them individually.

False Fingernails
These are sold in sets, one for each fingernail, in various lengths and shapes. There is also a process, best done professionally, of

wrapping the tips to extend them or of adding an acrylic substance that hardens and is then filed into shape and painted. Either method is excellent for one or two broken nails, or for those who have problems getting their nails to grow at all.

Foundation
This is merely another term for base or 'make-up'.

Hand Cream
This is an essential lubricant to prevent the hands drying and ageing prematurely. It should be used every time hands have been immersed in water and dried.

Highlighter
This is one of a girl's most valuable make-up accessories. Shiny, pearlized, iridescent, full of gold or silver – whether they are liquid, powder or cream, they bring life to the face when applied with care on places such as browbones and cheekbones.

Kohl
This is a powder used by Ancient Egyptians and Greeks not only for painting lines around eyes but also for darkening eyebrows and lashes. North African kohl is still a powder applied to the inner rims of the eyes with a rod. The Indian equivalent is a cream called kajal. Modern cosmetic products called kohl are usually in pencil form, in many colours and meant for colouring the inner rims of the eyes.

Lip Barrier
This is an emollient stick, often containing sunscreen, used to moisturize and prevent lips chapping.

Lip Colour
Lipsticks, lip pencils and lip gloss are all kinds of lip colour. All three add colour, lipsticks usually matt or frosted, lip pencils helping the

drawing of a clean outline and lip gloss adding shine, transparent or tinted.

Make-up Remover and Cleanser
It is vital to the continuing good condition of your skin that make-up is removed thoroughly; these items, with a special version for eye make-up, are essential.

Mascara
This is colour, found either in cake form, which is applied to the lashes with a brush and water, or in a creamy wand with its own applicator. The creamy varieties sometimes contain filaments which adhere to the lashes, making them appear thicker. All mascaras should make lashes look darker, thicker and more luxuriant; to achieve this, it is much better to apply several coats, separating the lashes carefully between each coat so they don't get clogged.

Mirror
Many people find a large hand mirror with a magnifier one side enormously helpful, particularly for plucking eyebrows and applying eye make-up. In any case, a large mirror surrounded by good even light is essential if your make-up isn't going to look uneven.

Nail Pencil
This is a pencil filled with white which cleans the tips of the nails and makes them look much brighter, when coloured polish isn't being worn.

Nail Polish
Also called varnish or enamel, nail polish is found in every colour of the rainbow from transparent to blood red, purple and black. It is best applied in several thin coats and allowed to dry completely in between.

Orange Sticks

These are used for gently pushing back cuticles and helping cuticle cream to penetrate underneath – a good trick is to round the edge with a penknife to soften it. They are helpful too in cleaning up smudges of polish when you've finished your manicure or pedicure.

Pencil Sharpeners

Now that so many eye, cheek and lip colours come in pencil form (from slim to chunky), it's vital to have them sharp at all times to make sure the wood doesn't snag the skin. So, keep sharpeners of the right size in your make-up bag – and clean the blade with surgical spirit.

Powder

Face powder comes in many tints but is most popular now in a colourless translucent form, used to 'set' make-up not to add colour. Keep loose powder on the dressing-table and carry a compact of pressed powder around with you.

Sponges

These are used for applying cream or stick foundation – they should be dampened first. Tiny sponge-tipped applicators for eyeshadow are also useful.

Tweezers

These are essential for keeping eyebrows tidy. Only pluck from below and be careful not to take out too many hairs at once – eyebrows add a great deal of character to the face and it's easy to overdo it.

Zinc

This is used in medicated lip ointments.

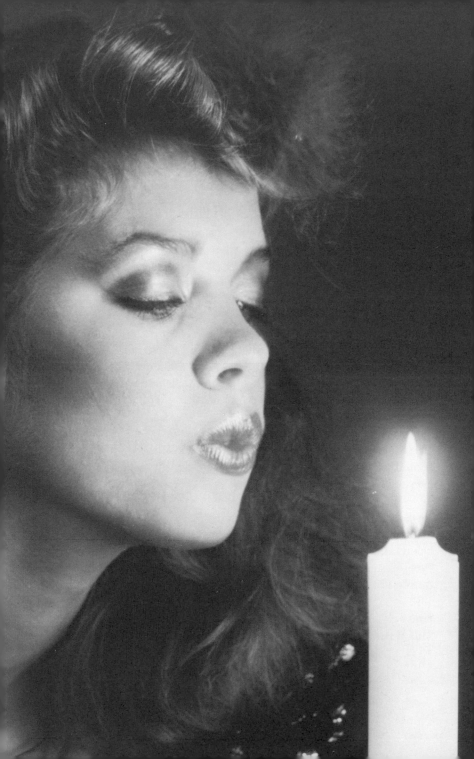

The Right Light:
What a Difference It Makes

The right light is vital to successful make-up. Light can play strange tricks with its strength and shadows and this can be used to your advantage provided you are aware of it. Blinking disco lights can do wonderful, strange things to the colours and contours of your face; you can use bright glittering colours to great effect – but beware of looking grotesque; soft candlelight is the most flattering of all, throwing flickering shadows and a mellow smoothness that few faces possess on their own; clear daylight can be soft or, with bright sun, very harsh.

The important thing is to accept the basic structure of your face and make the most of it. Make-up tricks to change its shape or contours must never be obvious or they create no illusion and lose their point.

Light changes colours, affects tone and depth. It also changes shape. A trick of the light can make an older face look younger or vice versa. Photographers can flatter their subjects with a light that smooths out lines or choose one that records every blemish. The same make-up will look different in daylight, sunlight, twilight or nightlight.

In summertime or in bright sunshine, pale colours look stronger and many people look best with no foundation – just a moisturizer or sunscreen plus very light eyeshadow, mascara, lip gloss (blusher for pale faces only). Nightlight needs stronger make-up. Start with moisturizer, then foundation to even the skin tone, outline lips with a pencil and dust over lots of loose face powder – the trick here is to use much more than you would expect and to dust off the excess; this way the matt look lasts longer. Next, contour your face with a powder blusher – use a darker shade in the hollows of the cheeks, perhaps around the eyes and temples. Shine on the eyes and lips reflects nightlight, makes the eyes look bright; also use lots of mascara and a dark pencil in the sockets and around the lashes for definition. Even a bright lip colour can fade away at night so give your mouth a sharp outline with the pencil. Experiment with an iridescent highlighter, turning your head to see how it catches the light and where it is most flattering to you – the centre of the eyelid, the browbone, down the bridge of the nose, cheekbones, in the crease of the upper lips, the cleft of the chin are good places to try.

Electric light is incandescent, very even, and you need definite colours ... real reds for lips, russet, soft green or blue for eyes.

Neon light is harsh; avoid pale lips and greys and browns which hollow out the cheeks. Choose warm tones: tangerine, shocking pink, gilded, pearlized corals. Outline the edge of your lips, and try iridescent rose, bronze or copper around the eyes.

Candlelight is most flattering, providing you're not sunburned. Avoid orange lips, hard eyes. Shape your face softly. Use lots of blusher. Soften, blush, lengthen the eye. For lips try muted blue-reds or wine shades and matt mauve, prune or grape for eyes.

The first essential is to see your face in the right light. Make up in the light you are going to be seen by, if at all possible. If you are going out in daylight, try and apply your make-up in the nearest equivalent – take a good mirror to a window, prop the mirror against it so that all the light falls on your face. Don't choose harsh direct sunlight or you may be tempted to use too heavy a hand and end up looking over made-up. For evenings, make up by electric light – then check the effect in softer light, candlelight, for instance, or a lower watt bulb. Place yourself in electric light in the same way as daylight – at a dressing-table or in a bathroom, for instance – and try and arrange light to fall on your face from all angles (side lights slightly in front of you and any overhead light falling on your face, not the back of your neck). Don't make up in bad light and, above all, don't make up where the source of light only falls on one side of your face. This will only mean your make-up ends up looking uneven or lop-sided.

Make sure you are comfortable and try and leave more than enough time for the job so that you are relaxed and don't run the risk of making time-consuming mistakes. First pin hair out of the way to expose your face – if you are using heated rollers or setting it in any way, this is a good moment to save time. Make sure your skin is scrupulously clean, then apply a moisturizer. It's a good idea to leave it a while to sink in, otherwise your foundation may slip around too much. Use this time to assemble all the colours you are planning to use before starting – this avoids the sudden discovery of a missing favourite lip or eye colour on which your whole make-up idea was based and the necessity of starting all over again.

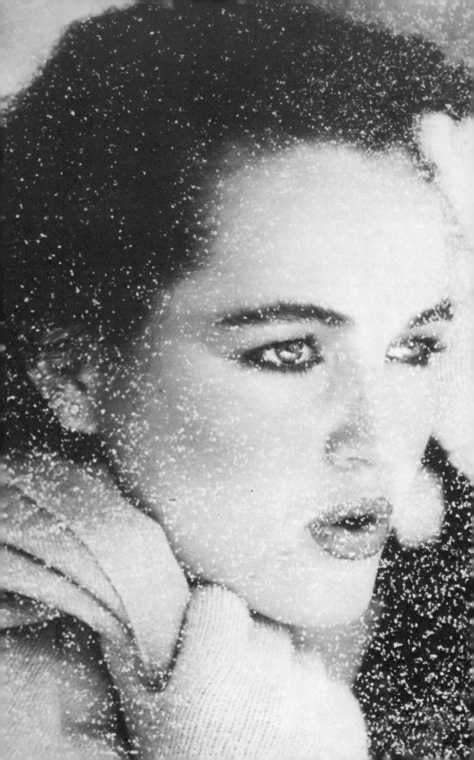

The Weather:
How It Affects Your Looks

How do you make your looks weather the weather? No one wants their make-up to run when the temperature soars, their hair to look a mess when the humidity is rising or the sun to make their skin resemble a peeled chestnut. Travelling, for most people, means more time in the sun or outdoors and although a bit of tan makes almost everyone look more vital and alive, over-exposure to sun is something you pay for with toughened, parched skin that will age faster, and dry brittle hair. These tips should help you plan your travelling beauty bag so that you look great wherever you are.

When it's winter – at home or abroad – protect skin from rain and cold. If you're a soap-and-water person, switch to a milder soap, less frequent washing and consider using a cream cleanser as an alternative. Don't wash your face immediately before going out in the cold – it's too drying and you risk chapping. Do it at least half an hour before and let the moisturizer sink in well. Cold reduces the elasticity of the skin and less humidity in the air makes for dryness, so you need to pay more attention to moisturization, which provides a protective barrier between the skin and the elements. Cold-weather activities – skiing, skating or a brisk walk – may work up a sweat and so increase chances of skin chapping. Lips need protecting; make sure the area around mouth and chin is well moisturized. Moisturizer should contain a good effective sunscreen. Sunglasses should be worn to prevent squinting in bright light, which encourages lines. Moisturizing glossy lip colours are the ones to look for and apply over a sunproofed lip protector and waterproof mascara.

In summer, your metabolism is speeded up and oil glands are more active, so change your moisturizer to something light and apply a sunscreen every morning before you make up. Try a tinted sunscreen to give you a healthy glow, with just mascara and lip colour.

Long-distance travellers often notice their nails become brittle, skin becomes very dry or unusually greasy, hair becomes oily. A lot of problems encountered by air-travellers are caused by dehydration en route – this can be counteracted by drinking lots of water during the trip. Take a nail strengthener and cuticle cream with you – a long air journey offers a terrific opportunity for a really good manicure – and lots of moisturizing hand cream. And, take a mild shampoo and a separate conditioner so that you can wash your hair as often as it needs and regulate your conditioning to the climate.

Be aware that the condition of your skin will change as climate changes. A cleanser or moisturizer that works in warm weather may not be rich enough in winter; if you go by plane, take some with you and apply during the journey.

You'll find *humidity plus air pollution* in cities like Rome, New York, Tel Aviv and Tokyo and you may find your skin looks dingy and your make-up fades as soon as you put it on. Air pollution can cause eye irritations that give you a puffy red-eyed look.

Use a good eyedrop designed to reduce redness, then lie down and apply cotton pads saturated with witch-hazel to your eyes. If you can put the witch-hazel in the refrigerator to cool it, it's especially refreshing. And, if witch-hazel isn't immediately to hand, try slices of cucumber or potato – old-fashioned remedies, but effective.

In cities like New York, for instance, the combination of cold, dry outdoor air and hot dry indoor air is very hard on skin and make-up. Dry skin can chap and develop an uneven texture. If you can, invest in a humidifier for indoors, use a richer moisturizer, and use

Patrick Demarchelier

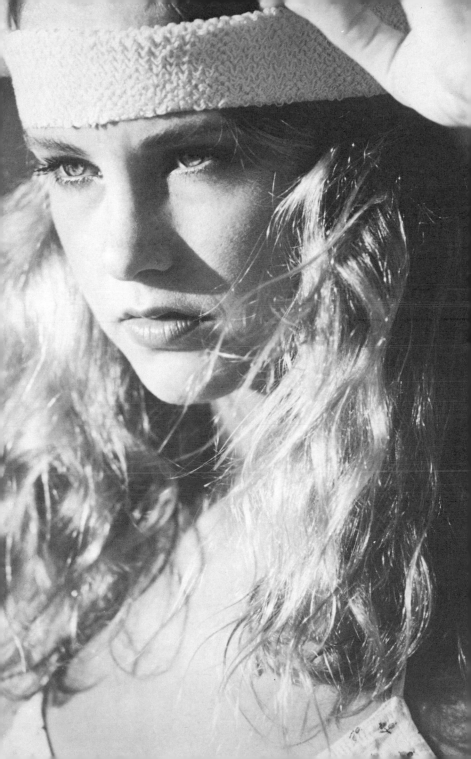

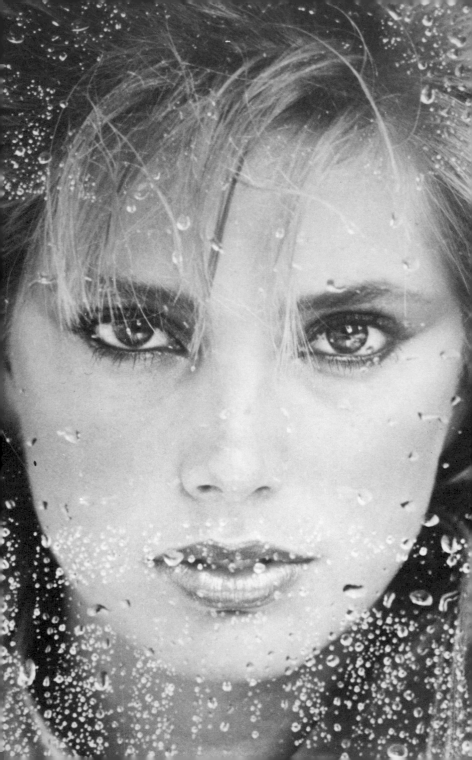

a moisturizing foundation with good coverage to add a protective barrier.

You'll find *very dry and hot weather* in places like Marrakesh, Baalbeck, the Gulf and on the Nile. Your lips may become parched and cracked and you'll probably have trouble making make-up go on smoothly. Laugh lines may seem more prominent. The big enemy to your looks in this environment is sun and, of course, its effects are intensified in the summer months. Protect your hair with a scarf, your skin with effective sunscreens and choose cream varieties of eye colour, blusher and moisturizing lipsticks.

You'll find *tropical heat and humidity* in Bangkok, Fiji or the Seychelles, for instance, and you may feel your make-up is melting as soon as you've put it on. The increased heat and humidity cause oil glands to be more active and the oil to be more fluid, so that it mixes with perspiration more. This tends to cause break-outs and unexpected rashes. Choose a foundation formulated for oily skins – this will help the rest of your make-up stay on your skin too – or try using a bronze-tinted sunscreen to give your skin a sunny glow.

Take a soothing medicated lotion to treat spots and a camouflage stick for dry blemishes. You'll probably find that powder eyeshadows and blushers stay on best; choose lipsticks with staying power and matt textures, slicking gloss on top to lighten the effect.

Expert Make-up for Different Skin Colourings

Very fair skins and spun-sugar silvery blond hair, epitomized by Scandinavian good looks, need the greatest possible care in make-up. The skin tends to be delicate, often very sensitive and dry and must always be protected from the sun. Moisturizer is essential at all times and should always be used under foundation. Only the lightest foundation is needed to achieve a smooth creamy texture which is the first step to porcelain pink-and-white looks; alternatively a gel make-up gives a tinge of honey colour that is very attractive but almost impossible to acquire safely from the sun. A light hand is the golden rule for fair good looks – experiment with almost any colour you like, but stick to the lightest shades.

The prettiest natural look for daytime is to make the most of the eyes, shadowing them in neutral colours that blend with the eyes, intensifying with kohl and mascara, shining lips with gloss, and just a hint of blush. In the evening a beautiful purity can be the answer – rose pink lips and cheeks, grey eyes highlighted with pink and gold, for instance.

Natural blondes, and particularly *dark blondes*, often have a lot of red in their hair colour; their skin tends to burn easily and freckle, like redheads. But they can take stronger colours than the very fair and have more choice than redheads. They are often considered

On the following eight pages are illustrations of suggested make-ups for different colourings.

Judi Bowker by Snowdon

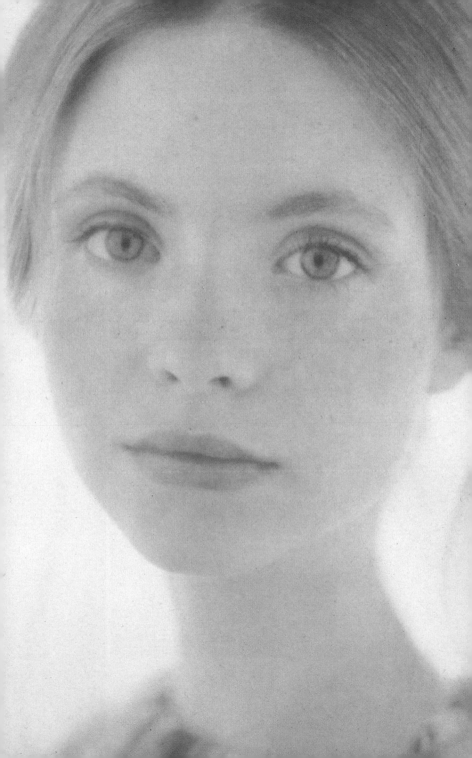

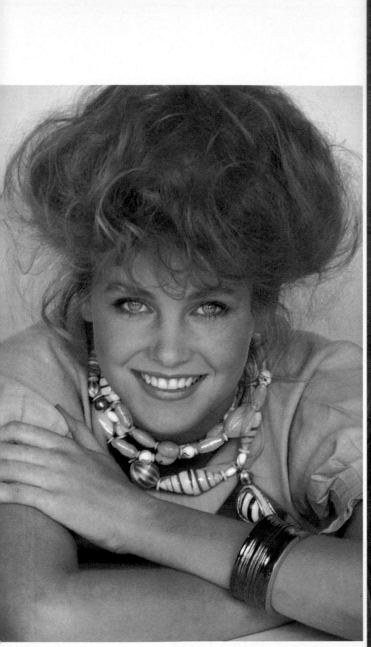

▲ Patrick Demarchelier

Albert Watson ▶

overleaf Lothar Schmid

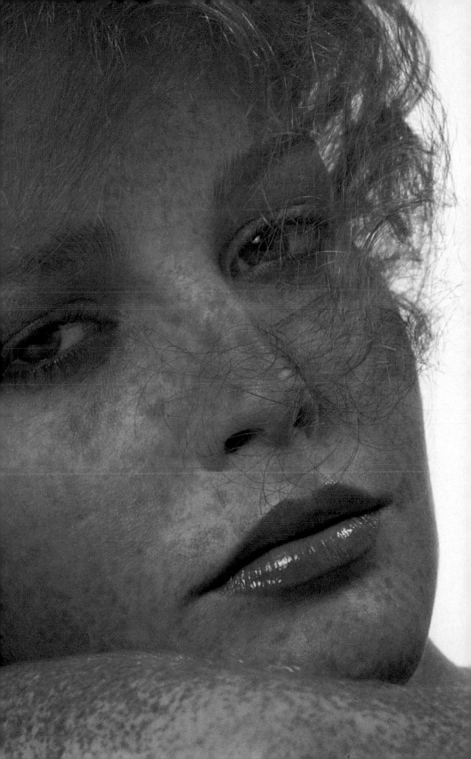

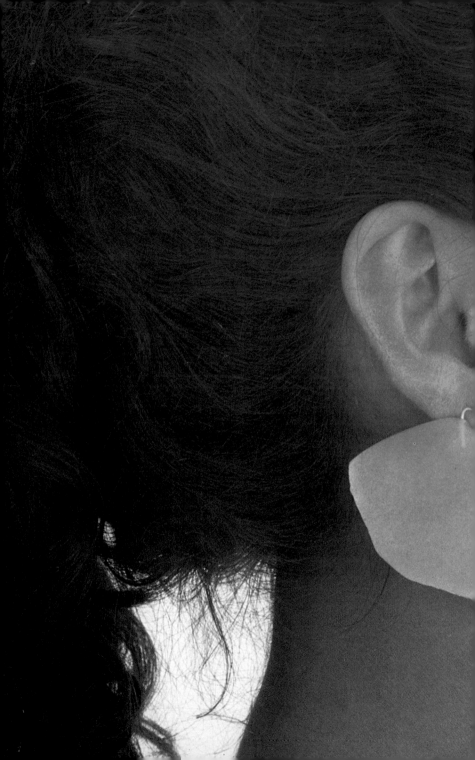

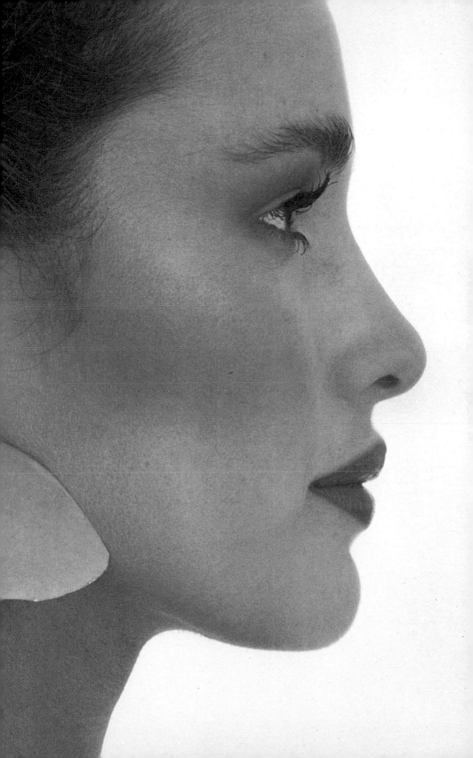

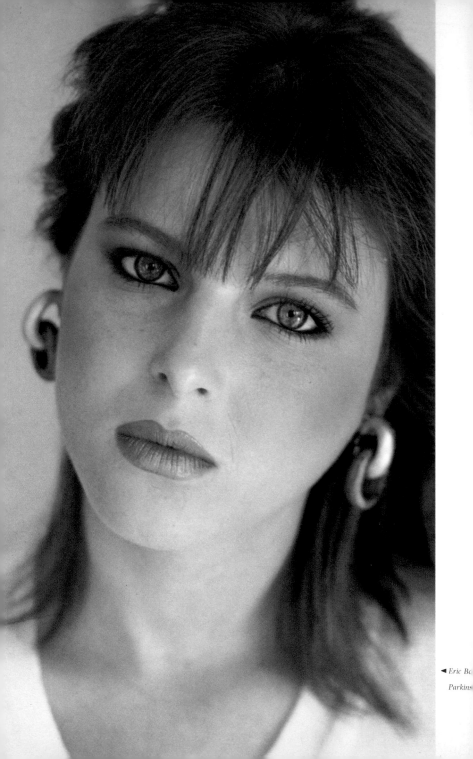

◄ Eric Bc
Parkins

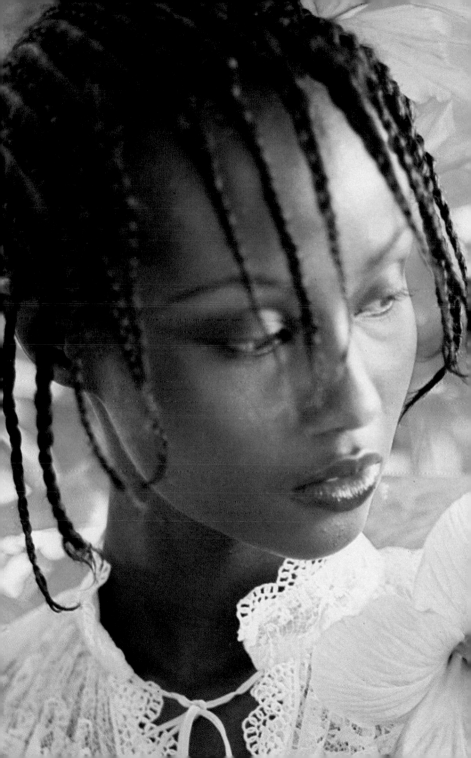

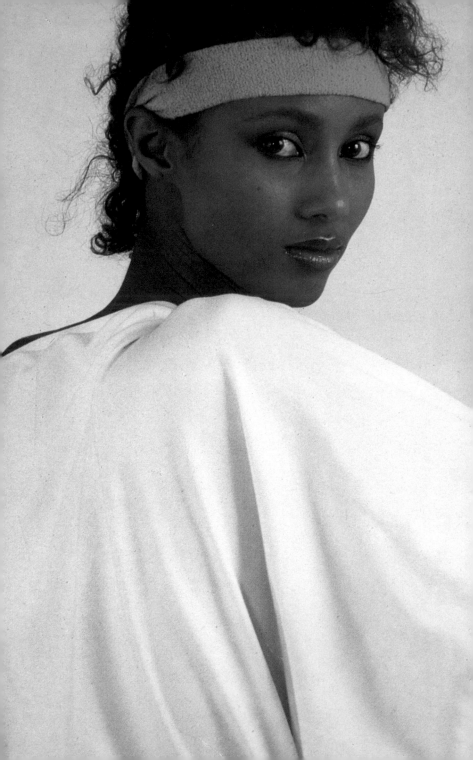

the lucky ones – any colour looks good on them. However, their skin is likely to be on the dry side and they should be careful using strong colours as their make-up should never be harsh.

It's easy to look washed-out wearing bright colours, but if you're fair-skinned and blond, be careful not to look over made-up. Choose a light-textured foundation (which allows your skin to show through) in a shade nearest your skin tone (test on the side of your jaw and choose in good daylight). Smoky colours – plum, grey, green, blue – look good around the eyes; use a pink to plum blusher and true pink or real red lipsticks.

Redheads with their tendency to beautiful translucent skin often have freckles too. The skin only has a small amount of melanin (the pigment that turns skin brown) in it and this means they burn easily or acquire freckles, which come from irregular pigmentation. Freckles don't appear only on the face but often all over the body – particularly across the shoulders. All freckles tend to fade during the winter but return as soon as the sun shines on the skin again. You can't stop them appearing, but a really good sunscreen will minimize them.

The best make-up results will come from learning to love your freckles and make the most of natural healthy colouring – only covering up for a specific smooth look in the evening. Freckles can be a terrific asset – many girls paint on fake ones for a healthy effect – so use a bronze gel base or just a moisturizing sunscreen during the day and a more covering foundation in the evening if you like.

With very pale, almost white eyelashes, it's worth considering having them dyed from time to time. Most salons do this, requiring a patch test twenty-four hours in advance to make sure you have no bad reaction; it is quite simple and makes a great difference to your looks. Otherwise, use lots of coats of mascara.

Natural colours for cheeks and lips are the tawny shades – peach, sienna, copper, bronze and terracotta – with rust, green and apricot tones around the eyes. Iridescents are great in the evening and gold is the redhead's natural highlighter, but stay away from silver. If you want to be more adventurous, play up either eyes *or* lips with a surprise colour but not both at once. Try violet or orchid pink around the eyes, shocking pink or raspberry lips.

Orientals often have creamy skin (with the tone ranging from pale ivory to warm olive) and black hair. This can look wonderful with really strong bright lips and smudgy charcoal eyes.

Brunettes with olive skin may find a mauve tinted moisturizer helpful in reducing any sallowness in the skin and often look best in earth tones for lips and cheeks – the darker your skin the more dramatic the colour can be; paler skins should stick to a softer look. Try green, bronze, brown around the eyes and highlight with creamy gold.

Girls with dark skins and dark brown or black hair often complain their skins are greasy and their make-up too shiny. This normally begins to disappear in their thirties, but then the danger is that the skin often goes very dry and, if neglected or not cleaned meticulously, may develop a grey or ashy look.

Dark skins need little or no tinted foundation or powder as they usually have a natural bloom and good all-over tone, but, if patchy, make-up can help to even out the tone; often a gel-bronze foundation is all that is needed. Red or yellow tints of foundation are not usually flattering – cool brown and earthy shades are best – and the gel or liquid varieties rather than stick or cream are usually most satisfactory.

Blushers in brick or wine shades (it's usually better to avoid light pink or red) and lipsticks in earth tones or wine are most becoming. Girls with the lighter types of brown skin can look wonderful with the brilliance of a true red or cyclamen pink. Pearlized lipsticks are inclined to make a mouth look larger; well-defined mouths usually look best with a minimum of colour, just glossed.

For eye make-up, avoid pearly colours if lids or the eye area is at all puffy. Where lids are narrow, a pearlized gel can help to shape the lid. If lashes are on the short side, a narrow band of cream or bone colour on the lid can give the illusion of more length. Kohl on the inner rims is very effective, as is lots of mascara. Good colour palettes to choose from are green through copper and bronze to golden brown and deep blue through plum to smoky grey.

Black skins have many variations in shade from mahogany to almost black; and normally tend to be oily. But, if exposed to a cold climate, many black skins suffer from dryness too. These complexions can burn in the sun, though not as severely as paler skins. Well-conditioned black skin should appear smooth and burnished and of an even tone – a greyish sheen means it's suffering from dryness or the wrong shade of foundation is being used.

Foundations and powders formulated for white skins are often not suitable for black, because they contain ingredients to deposit the greyish sheen mentioned above or a too red or too yellow tone. Many black skins, because of their oily texture, suffer from enlarged pores and, if exposed to cold and suffering from dryness, need moisturizing protection. Therefore, the choice of foundation is a vital one for successful make-up – a tinted moisturizer or bronzing gel may give just the right amount of coverage to protect and even out the skin tone, but if a heavier coverage is required, the base must be selected with great care. Most cosmetic ranges have dark shades of foundation and powder specially formulated for black skins, and there are cosmetic ranges specifically for black girls too.

The trick is to improve the natural polish of black skin. The use of highlighter (transparent white or a pink one with gold in it) above cheekbones, just above the upper lip, down the bridge of the nose and around the eye area is particularly effective. Use sparingly and let the natural skin show through the surface sheen. Transparency is the prettiest effect to aim at, no matter how much colour you choose to apply. Thin cheek gels in copper, wine or even magenta; and lip gloss, over a matt colour if you like, ranging from coral, brick, plum and brandy shades to the darkest wine and blackberry are good products to experiment with. For eyes, all the iridescent products are perfect – for a neutral make-up, shade in gold, apricot and rust, or amethyst, rose and burgundy, depending on the particular tone of your skin; for evening or for fun, try the peacock blues, greens, purples with silver or gold highlight. Add kohl pencil inside the lower rim and lots of mascara in several coats, separating the lashes as you go.

A good rule is to stay away from muddy colours and experiment with the clear vivid ones that look harsh on paler complexions.

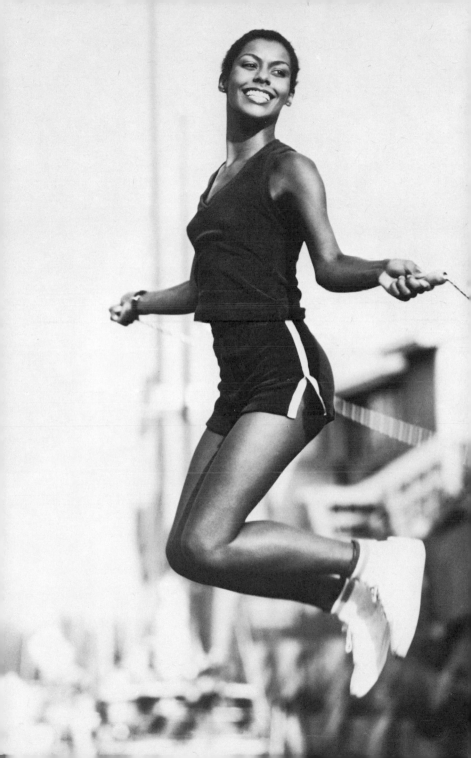

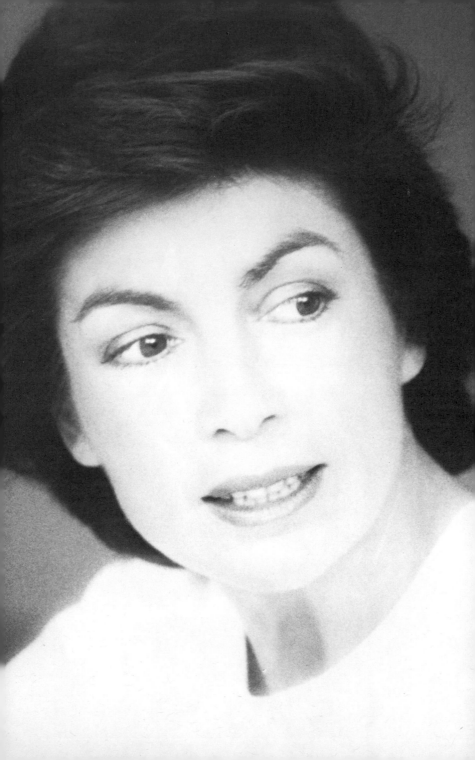

Expert Make-up for the Woman over Thirty-five

When forty starts approaching many women panic – they start rushing off to plastic surgeons to discuss face-lifts only to be told they are much too young and not to return for several years. Forty is *not* the beginning of the end; a few lines certainly don't mean the whole face is disintegrating; and a bit of overweight can be removed, even though it may take longer.

All that is really needed is a beauty reassessment, a re-think of make-up, hair style and colour. In order to maintain energy, healthy hair and skin, more attention must be paid to exercise and diet – the effects of years of careless diet and body neglect will start to show in the thirties; from then on, weight-control is much harder and it takes more effort and longer to improve skin and hair health.

The body needs more help to function efficiently; the skin is beginning to lose its elasticity, hair may lose its colour and texture, and make-up needs a different approach.

Around forty is when many women who have never had a skin problem in their lives discover the distress of specific forms of acne, psoriasis, blackheads, whiteheads and enlarged pores. Brown spots can appear and don't disappear – these can now be minimized by regular use of special fading creams. Skin colour can change or go patchy and this discolouration is often due to sluggish circulation – exercise or a brisk walk will improve the tone and a soft cream or fluid foundation in the correct shade will do the rest. If there are broken veins or blemishes to hide, use a camouflage cream or stick.

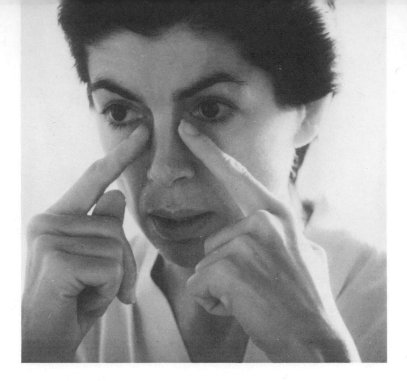

Aim to look well, rather than slavishly using the latest fashion colours to look trendy. A light hand with make-up is essential – heavy make-up is ageing, as are dark colours and hard lines.

Choose a foundation to improve your natural tone – perhaps with a little extra pink or peach in it. Avoid cool beiges unless you have a naturally high colour, in which case a mud beige will act as camouflage, and try a green tinted moisturizer underneath. Skin shouldn't look too powdered – or shine too much, although this is unlikely as most skins dry out as they get older. Too matt a finish looks lifeless, so be particularly careful not to use powdery make-up or powder under the eyes or on the area of the browbone. Powder sinks into every slight imperfection, is bad for delicate skin and makes the eyes look lifeless. Use translucent powder – a neutral colour or just a shade lighter than your foundation – and fluff it on

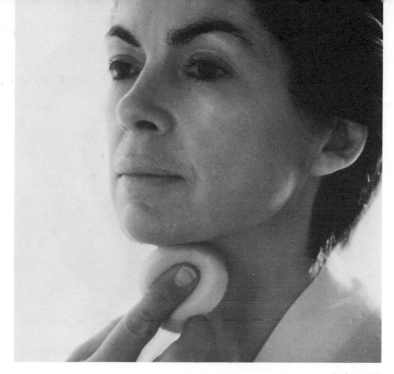

Sandra Lousada

very lightly with a puff. Be careful on lines running from nose to mouth – they are the first place foundation and powder sink into, giving a tired impression.

Use blusher sparingly – if it is very well blended it is flattering, but beware of adding to an already high skin tone and looking feverish.

Beware of iridescent eye make-up – shine can emphasize the smallest blemish. And avoid very bright colours; a shade several tones paler than your eye colour is often a good guide. The varieties of eyeshadow that are painted on with water (a dampened sponge-applicator) are often the most satisfactory as they last better and don't settle into the creases, although many of the newer cream formulas are excellent. Avoid dark eyeliners; use soft smoky green, blue or grey and smudge a line near the lashes.

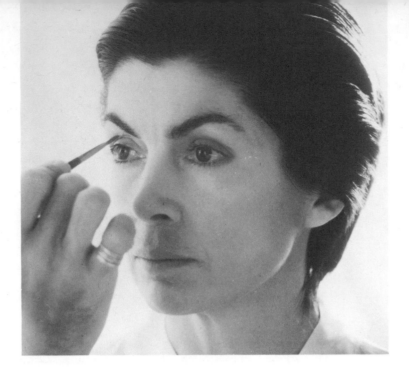

Don't be tempted by gold, silver or glitter – they will just draw attention to everything you are trying to minimize. Eyebrows need to be kept trim – neither too thin nor too prominent. Always pluck from below and never use a hard dark pencil. If your brows have thinned, use a soft grey or brown pencil and make light feathery strokes. Aim at keeping the whole eye area moist and soft-looking, neither too dry or powdery nor so shiny that the creases are very evident. If your eyelids tend to droop at the outer corner, keep eye-liner and shadow 'lifted', with slightly more depth of shadow towards the temple. Don't make obvious lines and don't extend the make-up beyond the corner of the eye unless it is very carefully blended. A touch of highlighter immediately below the brow is a good idea. So is mascara, but choose dark brown or grey rather than hard black. A special eye make-up remover is a good investment as it whisks away all the colour with minimum disturbance.

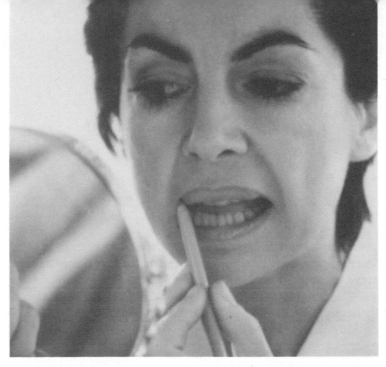

Sandra Lousada

Cream your lips at night to keep them soft and blot carefully before putting on lipstick. A good tip is to take your foundation over the edge of your lips, powder well, then outline with a lip pencil or lip brush, fill in with colour, blot again and powder again. This helps to maintain a clean outline and avoids the colour 'bleeding' into the tiny lines around the mouth. Choose a lipstick colour that is light and creamy.

Pinks, corals and light reds are most becoming – but it's worth experimenting with the plum shades. Pale lipstick will make the lips look dry, brighter ones add life to the skin and eyes. Iridescent colours will show up every tiny line – matt creamy shades, with just a touch of extra gloss if you like, are much more flattering.

If the mouth tends to droop at the corners, extend the outline of the lower lip upwards and don't take the colour on the top lip all the way into the corner.

Colour Co-ordination:
What to Wear with What

There are dozens of choices in terms of the colours you like to wear and the colours you put on your face. And the little thing that can make the most excitement and change in your looks is a new make-up colour – a new blusher, lipstick, eyeshadow or whatever. It doesn't mean you need a new make-up colour for every piece of clothing, but it does mean choosing your make-up within the spectrum of colours that suit your hair and skin tone *and* the colours you choose to wear, so that the overall effect is in harmony from top to toe. Each colour you choose to wear or put on your face should enhance the others and flatter your skin, hair and eyes. Sometimes it's fun to keep eyes, lips and cheeks the same colour as the dress you're wearing – pink, for instance – but this needs expert application to be really effective.

White, cream, beige, brown, grey, black – these are the neutral colours which suit almost everyone; make-up should then be in clear colours to flatter hair and skin. At night, gold and silver highlight is very effective with frosted lipsticks and cheek colours.

Yellow, orange, tan – these are sometimes difficult to wear as they are inclined to reflect on to the skin and give a sallow impression. They are good with a tan and redheads look wonderful in these colours – others are often wise to put white, cream, beige or grey between them and their face. Peach or tawny blushers work best, with peach, coral, vermilion, sienna and rust for lips. On eyes try moss green, bronze, golden or smoky browns – brown mascara is softer than black – and highlight in gold.

Green – from pale almond to forest, this is the natural colour for redheads but good on blondes and brunettes too, particularly anyone with hazel or green eyes. Green can make pale skins look paler, so it might be a good idea to use a warmer shade of foundation and make sure your blusher is in the apricot to tawny group. Try bois de rose, crimson, light red or russet lipstick and shade eyes with apricot and teal green, smoky greens, copper or try mauve with clear green kohl lining the inner rim.

Blue – from sky through violet to navy and purple, this is probably the most popular colour in the rainbow; some form suits almost everyone. Like green it can make pale skins look paler, so check your foundation shade. Russet or rose pink blusher looks pretty; for lips try all the pinks from pastel peach to shocking and magenta and true red. Don't try for a perfect match on your eyes, but keep them in the same family – the smoky blues and violets are more flattering than the light chalky shades – or try apricot, copper and brown.

Red – this cheers anyone up; a touch is often enough and could just be your lipstick. With bright red lips, keep eyes neutral – charcoal is great and bronze is interesting with red, if lips are pale and glossy.

Pink – this ranges from rose to fuchsia, crimson and wine. Light clear pinks are among the most flattering colours to wear, but when you get into the crimson and wine shades, be sure your make-up doesn't appear muddy. Choose clear bright lipsticks in the same family and pink cheeks; try grey, smoky blue, plum or orchid pink on the eyes and pink highlighter.

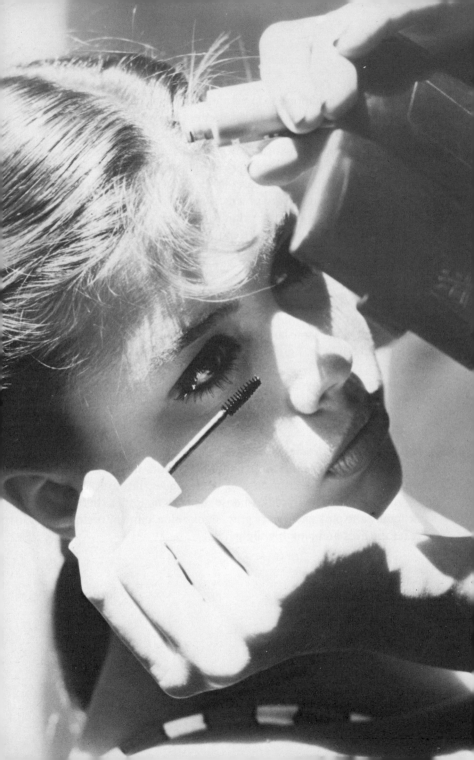

Your Face:
How to Change Its Shape

Play up your good points, minimize the bad and proceed with caution. Too often contouring and highlighting is done with a heavy hand and the result is grotesque, but with extreme care much can be done with make-up to improve the basic shape of your face, eyes or lips.

First, face your problems – look at yourself in a really good light and work out the shape of your face, what you like about it and what you don't. Next, look at your eyes – are they wide- or close-set? Narrow, protruding or too round? Do your lids droop or do your brows overhang? Are your eyebrows too heavy or an untidy shape? Now, your lips – are they too full, too narrow or uneven?

Take your face first and, using the principle of light and shade, decide what you are going to emphasize and what you want to diminish. The upper line of the cheekbone, the browbone, the temples, the ridge of the nose, the centre of the upper lip and the centre of the chin are all good places to try and highlight. A wide nose, heavy jaw and cheek hollows are places to experiment with shading – use a darker tone of foundation or one of the special contour powders or creams described as 'face-shapers'. With both light and shade, use very little to start with and build up until you achieve the effect you want; this will take some time and a lot of patience.

Now eyes. If they are wide-set you are fortunate, but if they are too close together they will appear farther apart if you apply a deep, smoky tone of shadow to the outer corners of the eyelid, blending

(Continued on page 232)

Changing the Shape
of Your Face

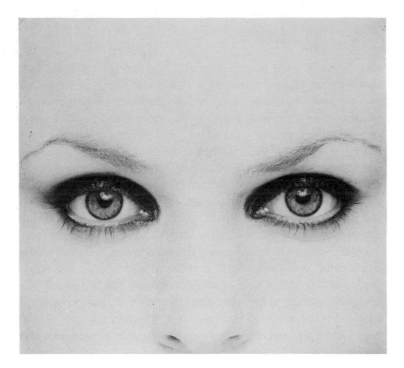

Widen Your Eyes
Eyes that have too much lid showing should be coloured across the entire lid, into the crease and halfway across lower lid and then blended as shown.

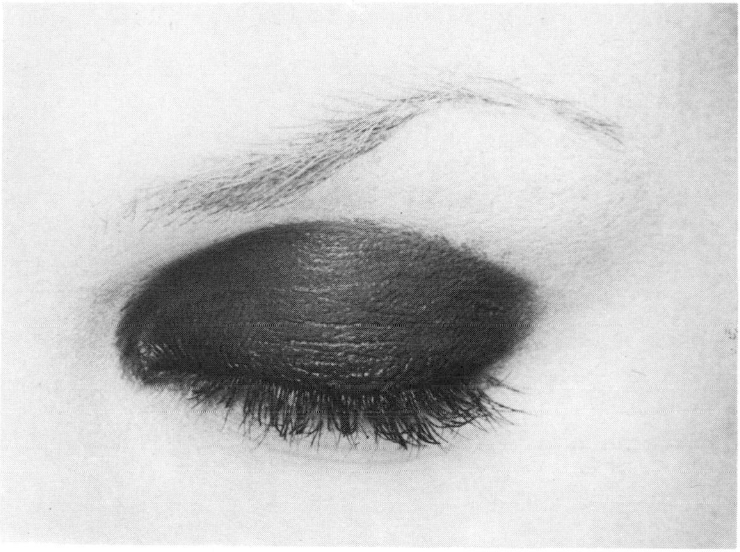

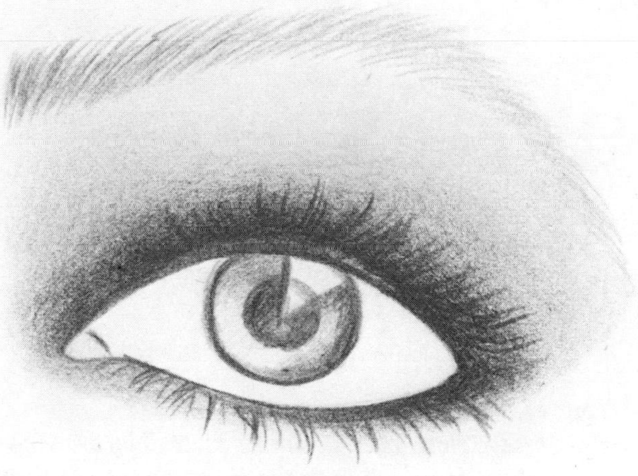

Photographs by John Swannell,
drawings by Barbara Daly

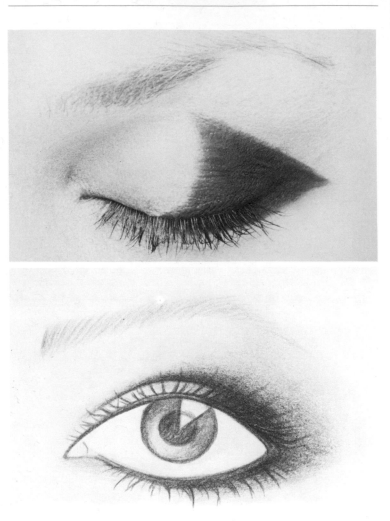

Widen Your Eyes
Eyes that are set too close together can be widened by drawing a triangular shape with an eye pencil from the outer corners, halfway across both upper and lower lids and crease. Then blend as shown.

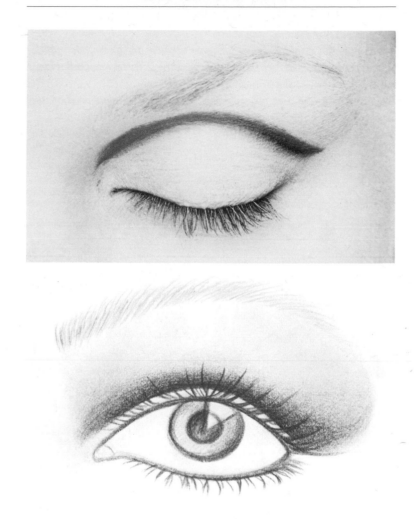

Open Your Eyes
Eyes with little lid showing and lots of space and bone need a light eyeshadow on the lid, a dark line drawn in the crease then blended up and out.

Reshape Your Face

To slim the bridge of your nose take a paintbrush and a cream foundation about three shades deeper than your skin tone and draw a small triangle at the inner end of the brows. Blend carefully.

To slim the lower part of your nose, paint a small elongated triangle vertically above the nostrils, then blend carefully.

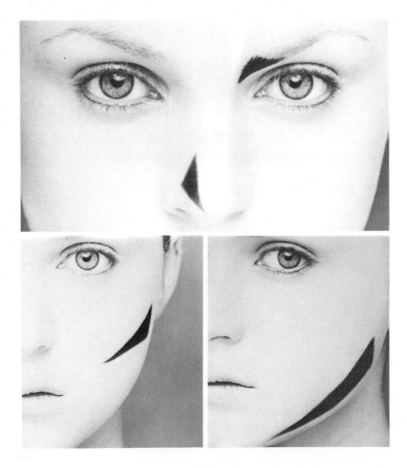

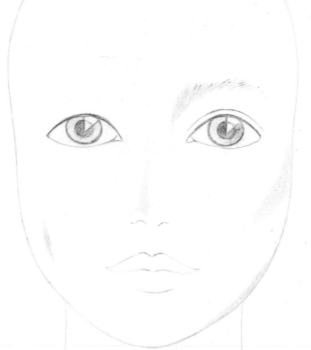

To slim the jawline, paint a long wedge shape just above the edge then blend carefully. Use a cream foundation about three shades darker than your skin, but not a red tone. To raise the cheekbones, draw elongated triangles just below the bones, fill in and blend.

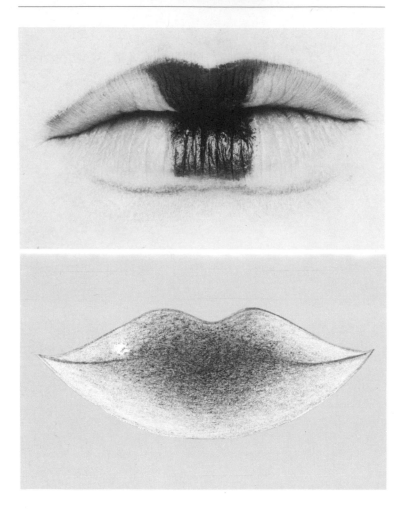

Balance Your Lips

If your lips are too full take a lip pencil and outline the centre of the top lip, then fill in the centre section of both lips, with a darker colour lipstick than your chosen shade. Blend as shown in drawing.

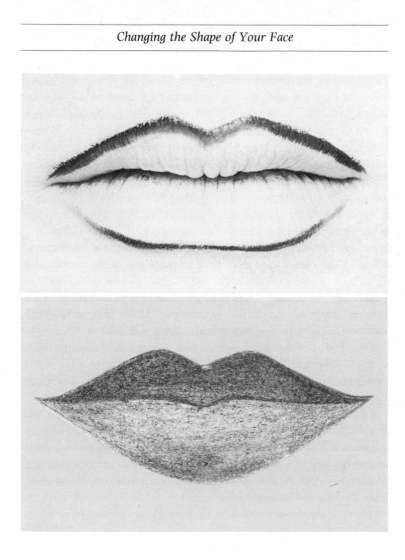

If your upper lip is narrow, paint a line with a pencil just over the top lip edge, fill in the upper lip with lipstick, and use a lighter shade on lower lip.

it up towards the end of your eyebrow and just under the lower lashes. If they are narrow, try applying dark shadow close to the lashes, from the centre of the lower lashes round the outer corner across the top to the inner corner. Smudge for a soft effect. If eyes protrude, they will appear less prominent if you draw a band of colour right round the eye close to the lashes in a medium to deep shade. A pencil is good for this; smudge it lightly so the line isn't too hard. If eyes are too round, elongate them by shading two thirds of the upper lid (the outer section) and blending it upward to the brow and just under the outer corner.

Droopy lids will appear less sleepy if colour follows the natural shape of the eye; widen the band towards the outer corner and blend it outwards and upwards, with a little colour under the eye for balance. Overhanging brows can be lifted if you apply shadow from the inside corner of the eye over the top lid, then around the outer corner and bottom lid; smudge for a soft outline.

If you feel your eyebrows are too heavy and decide to pluck them yourself, take great care not to overdo it and remove a lot of the character from your face. Never pluck the top line and never cut them – only pluck from below, a few hairs at a time.

If you feel your eyebrows are too thin and sparse or too pale, use an eyebrow pencil. If it is depth you need, choose a brown or grey colour, but if it is just added line that's required, choose a colour to match your own brows. Either way, start near the bridge of the nose and work outwards, using soft feathery strokes and extending them slightly at the outer edge.

Lips that are too full will look smaller if you use a light shade of lipstick and concentrate the colour on the centre section. Thin lips will look fuller if the outline is drawn *just* outside the edges and they are filled in with colour and gloss. Uneven lips can be better balanced if two tones of colour, plus gloss, are used – use the lighter tone and gloss on the narrow lip and leave the fuller one darker and matt. Lips that droop at the corners and give a sad expression can be tilted by extending the outline of the lower lip at the corners.

Barry Lategan

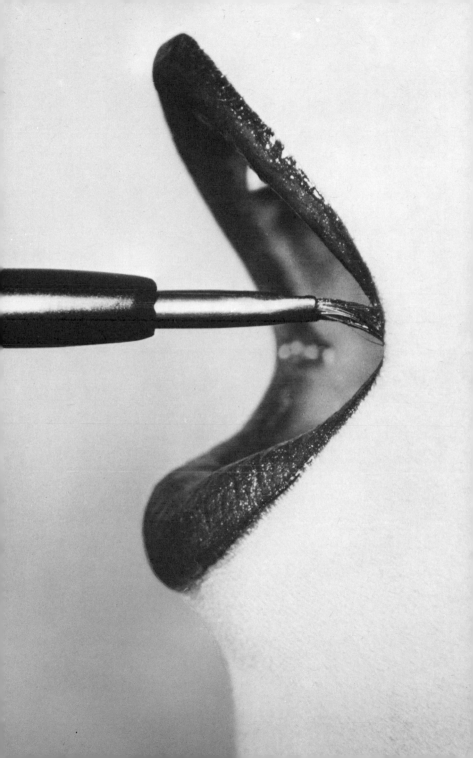

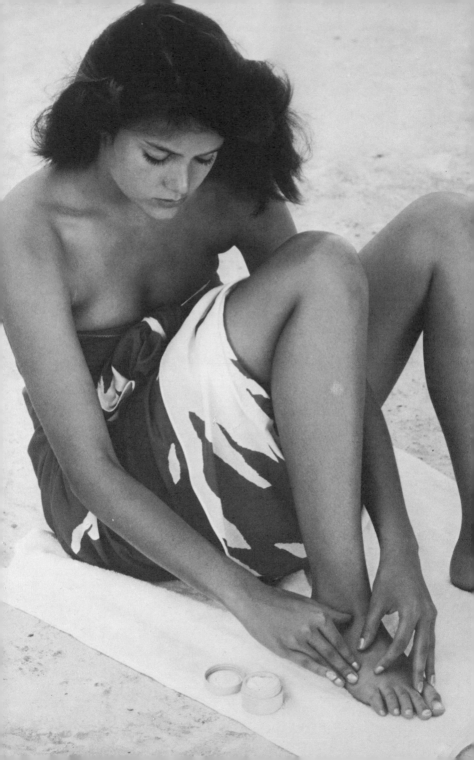

Hands and Feet:
How to Add the Final Touch

Beautifully kept hands, soft and smooth with strong well-shaped nails all one length are quickly noticed. Equally quickly noticed are dry, blistered, wrinkled ones with bitten, dirty or split nails. In summer or on holiday, feet are exposed to the same sort of scrutiny and toenails are as noticeable as fingernails, needing just as much year-round care.

Feet work enormously hard for their living – they take the full weight of your body and their condition can affect the way you feel each day. Everyone knows the facial expression (and feel) of pain that comes from ill-fitting shoes, corns, blisters or just feet that have walked too far and aren't used to it. Problem feet can be due to a variety of causes, including heredity, ill-fitting shoes, poor posture and fatigue. Flat-footedness and a predisposition to bunions caused by the first toe being shorter than the second seem to be inherited. But many other problems are the result of foot abuse – expecting the foot to carry all kinds of weight in all sorts of footwear over all kinds of surface without any care or maintenance at all.

It's an excellent idea to have a professional manicure and pedicure from time to time, but in between set aside a regular hour or so at least once a week for hands and feet – and start with your feet because you'll need your hands to work on them; then they can rest and the polish can dry while you attend to your hands.

How to Choose your Nail Colour
First, examine carefully the shape of your hands, feet and the condition of your nails – but consider each separately.

First your hands – if you are fortunate enough to have been born with really beautifully shaped hands and fingers and have nourished and cared for your nails, you can choose virtually any colour of the rainbow as polish. They run from brown, russet and plum ... to the pale pretty pinks and shocking ... to the vibrant poster-paint primaries, blue, green, yellow ... and all the true brilliant reds. If you have great nails, polish them bright.

The very pale, opaque, ivory or bone shades, and the harsh iridescent or very dark colours are more eye-catching than medium tones. So, if you feel your hands leave a bit to be desired in the way of shape but your nails are in good condition, choose mid-tone corals and pinks that blend naturally with your clothes and make-up.

But, however good or bad the shape of your hands, if your nails are broken, bitten or unsightly, forget colour and put your effort towards repairing them. Buff them to a natural shine – this also stimulates circulation, and blood feeds the matrix where the nail grows – or paint them with a clear natural polish which will help protect and strengthen them.

Tips to Remember when Painting Nails
The prettiest nail is filed into a soft oval, the cuticle massaged away and loosened off the nail, the skin kept soft with hand cream.

Start by filing nails, properly, with the fine side of an emery board, always towards the centre. Never file them into points or down into the corners.

If you paint the colour down the side of the nails, it tends to broaden their appearance, so only do this if they are long and narrow.

If nails incline to be broad, leave the last tiny strip on either side clear.

If nails are slim, they may look good with the moons left clear, but this also has a widening effect, so if they are the slightest bit square, cover the moons.

If you decide on half-moons, the first stroke of colour should be taken across from one side of the moon's edge to the other; they need a very steady hand for a good effect, so unless you've had plenty of practice, leave it to a professional manicurist.

Before you start painting, be sure your nails are absolutely clean – after removing obvious dirt, a white pencil run under the nail tip brightens the tone.

For soft nails, or those that are flaking, a nail hardener will help and a base coat or protective top coat will lengthen the life of your chosen nail colour.

The best way to remove old polish is to wet a cotton pad with remover, hold it on the nail for a minute to pre-soften the polish and wipe off slowly. Then, most important, wash hands and around nails thoroughly to take off the remover.

A weekly manicure is plenty; too frequent use of remover weakens your nails' natural strength. Remover is largely acetone and excessive use of it can cause the essential cementing ingredients to dry out, which causes splitting nails. It's better to touch up polish between manicures rather than remove it every time there's a chip. Buy oil-based remover – it's less drying.

Putting on Polish

Prime with a base coat to prevent chipping. Allow it to dry, then apply several coats of polish, drying each coat before applying the next. Last, put on a top coat for added strength. Delicate nails can benefit from nail hardeners applied to just the free, unattached edge.

Apply polish with decisive strokes from the base of the nail to the tip – make sure you don't get too much polish on the brush or you will get blobs on the nail and be tempted to go back and smooth them out. Three thin coats will give a much smoother result than one thick one – and will last much longer.

The bright, vivid shine of polish is a nice finishing touch for toenails, especially in summer – or whenever you wear sandals.

Pick a good basic colour that will go with many things, so you won't have to change polish too often. Polish should last two weeks.

Again foot condition, foot shape and the health of their nails must influence your choice of colour, but generally speaking a bright clear red, rust or magenta looks prettiest. With open-toed shoes or sandals, don't forget that your feet are very much a part of your top-to-toe appearance and the colour of your toenails should blend or contrast deliberately with the colours you are wearing.

Twelve Steps to a Professional Pedicure
First assemble your equipment – most of these things last quite a long time and are useful for your manicure or other parts of your beauty routine, so it's not such a daunting, expensive list as it may first appear:

nail polish remover, cottonwool, tissues, a bowl large enough for both your feet to rest in comfortably when filled with warm, soapy water (a mild shampoo is ideal, don't use detergent), a towel, nail brush, pumice stone, emery board, orange sticks, cuticle cream or oil, body lotion, base coat, coloured polish, top coat.

Procedure

1) Remove all traces of existing polish.

2) Soak both feet in the bowl of soapy water for about five minutes (while you are doing this, you can use the time to remove old polish from your fingernails).

3) Use pumice stone on soles, heels and sides of feet to remove rough dry skin.

4) Dry feet carefully, particularly between the toes.

5) Apply cuticle cream or oil around the toenail and massage well. Then, using a rounded orange stick (reshape and soften the ends with a penknife and make sure there are no splinters to catch and tear your skin), gently push back the cuticles and help the

cream or oil to penetrate underneath and reach the matrix where the nails form and grow.

6) Rinse feet in warm clear water and dry again thoroughly.

7) Clip nails straight across; don't clip into the side or try to cut a curved shape as this encourages in-growing toenails, which are unsightly and painful. (Toenails shouldn't be too long or they will press against your shoes, but they should be all one length.)

8) File the ends smooth with an emery board. Massage toes and feet well with a moisturizing body lotion, then wipe the nail area clean with a tissue (polish won't stick if any greasiness is left.)

9) Twist tissue into two long sausage shapes and wind them in and out of your toes – this separates the toes and prevents polish smudging from one toe to the other.

10) Apply base coat – more important on toenails than fingernails as they tend to be rougher; this will provide a smooth foundation for polish.

11) Apply two coats of your chosen colour – and lastly a top coat if you wish. Allow each coat to dry between each application and let the final surface dry for at least half an hour when you've finished (about the time it takes to give yourself a manicure).

12) Lastly, massage well with body lotion again.

Manicure Repeat the process for pedicure, omitting the pumice stone and filing your nails into a gentle curve. Again, a shorter all-one-length shape is much prettier than varying lengths, so choose a medium length that you can maintain. Make-up or foundation for hands is not usually very satisfactory, except for photography, but there are fading creams to help minimize freckles or brown spots.

Just remember it is always better to wear no coloured polish at all than to go round with chipped or peeling finger- or toenails.

For a complete step-by-step description of a perfect manicure, see pages 72–5.

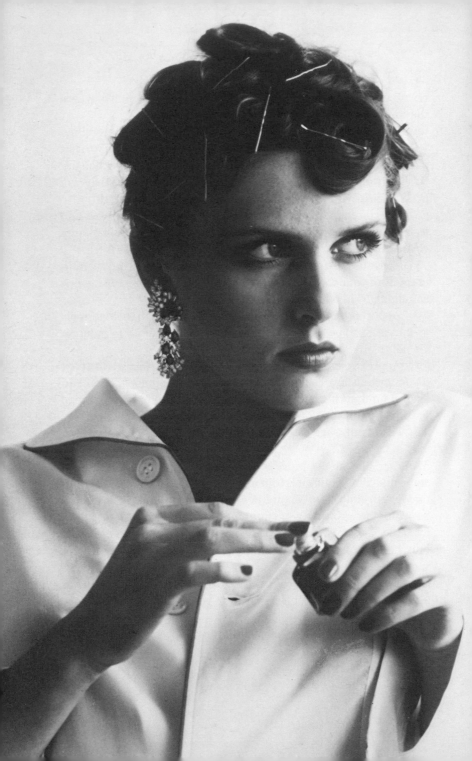

Scent:
How to Make the Most of Its Fragrant Aura

The right fragrance, worn constantly, sprayed or smoothed on from head to foot, is a powerful beauty asset. It enhances glowing skin, perfect make-up, shining hair and is truly the final touch to beauty. It's more evocative than any other sense – just a passing whiff evokes a nostalgia for past loves and pleasures or brings a feeling of fear or distress with such speed you are amazed.

It is a *vital* element in beauty, but also one of the most personal and individual. What you like on yourself, what you like on someone else and what others like on you *can* be one and the same scent but are much more likely to be three different fragrances. One of the most intriguing aspects is how scent reacts to skin – it smells of one thing in the bottle, another on immediate application, then as it warms up and involves the skin's chemistry, top, middle and base notes (as the various groups that form a blended perfume are called) begin to show their strength and the lasting, lingering fragrance that will be yours becomes apparent about half an hour later.

Body chemistry is as individual as fingerprints and however many costly ingredients go into one single fragrance, you, your skin, will add the final one. The oils, minerals and moisture secreted by glands below the skin's surface, plus the elements that form skin, are what will make one fragrance smell different on each member of a group of wearers.

What else changes fragrance? Smoking can reduce its lasting power, as can air pollution; internal or external medication can distort a scent; and where you apply it makes all the difference to its potency – the best places are pulse points where natural warmth will cause the scent to develop to its maximum level, but this needs some experimentation. Some women find the inside of the crook of the elbow is great; others find behind the knees, between the breasts, on the wrists, behind the ears or at the nape of the neck works best for them. All fragrance should be treated as an accessory – an essential one – that envelops you like the lightest silk shawl printed in a myriad of colours, trailing behind you as you walk ...

All great perfumes are complex interweavings of scented strands – hundreds become part of one overall blend, each one playing an important role in the final effect. Some are light and cool, some heavy and warm; some bright and fresh, some dark and sensuous. Some act as stimulants, some as narcotics (and poppies aren't the only flowers to have this effect), some refresh, some lull. Some send out quiet, but insistent messages on a deep, primeval level ... our sense of smell may be much less acute than other mammals', having been used less and less over the ages, but it is still keen enough to accept messages of attraction, disgust, reassurance or warning.

An expert 'nose', as the great perfume creators are called, can identify the main ingredients of a perfume but even with scientific help he will have trouble determining the exact quantities used in the final blend. And so the great scents retain their exclusivity. Many of these ingredients have been known and used since thousands of years before Christ – musk, sandalwood, camphor, myrrh and frankincense, for instance – and the word 'perfume' dates from the time when some ancient discovered, having walked through scented smoke, that the smell clung to his body and made him (or her) more attractive. Now there are synthetic equivalents for many of them and science has provided other interesting and long-lasting unidentifiable odours, but nothing really compares

with the real thing, which is becoming rarer all the time, account-
ing for the soaring high costs of perfume and fragrant products.

Some women like to find one scent that suits them and stick to
it for the rest of their lives, others like to change according to their
mood and others find it a good idea to change according to the
seasons (fresh, green fragrances for summer, warm, spicy ones for
winter) or climate.

Whatever your preference, scent should become a part of your
daily life. Don't think of it as something to wear only occasionally
or as the last thing you add before leaving the house. Learn to layer
it – splash on cologne or eau de toilette directly after a bath or
shower (after drying yourself!) and use matching scented soaps,
bath oil, powder and deodorant – then follow with the most concentrated version and use it sparingly. Your scent should be as
personal as your signature. The right one could be as simple as the
single scent of a herb or flower or it could be a complex mixture of
flowers, roots, spice, wood, leaves, moss, fruit and animal notes
(see below).

It's purely a matter of taste, yours and those around you, and to
help you choose, here is an A-Z of some of the terms used when
describing scent and a few of the main ingredients involved (cross-
references, especially of common words used in a technical sense,
are given in italic):

ABSOLUTE OR CONCRETE a pure concentrated oil distinguished
from an *essential oil* by the process through which it is obtained.
ALDEHYDE a synthetic fragrance and vital ingredient in modern
perfumery.
AMBERGRIS the spew of sperm whales goaded by indigestion and
found floating on the ocean or cast up on beaches, mostly in the
Indian Ocean or South Pacific. An unsurpassed *fixative* in perfume.
ANIMAL NOTES the natural *fixatives*: musk, civet, castoreum
(from the beaver) and ambergris.

BERGAMOT an oil obtained from a small green orange found in Southern Italy. A synthetic version is widely used now as the natural oil was found to cause brown patches on skin exposed to strong sunlight.

BOUQUET a mixture of smells; also the smell developing (as with wine) as it warms.

CIVET a glandular secretion from the civet cat, found in North East Africa and used as a *fixative*.

CHYPRE a particular type of perfume; opinions differ as to its definition and origin. The base contains oakmoss, labdanum (cistus), calamus and styrax, but to this are added *animal, fruity* or *floral notes*, giving many variations to this heady appealing type.

CITRUS an essence from the citrus fruit family: orange (the flower and the fruit), lemon, grapefruit, neroli and bergamot; or a type of perfume with strong citrus notes: the fresh *green* varieties and most eau de colognes.

CLASSICS a term often applied to the famous named perfumes, mostly pre-1940, but also referring to more modern ones that have become very popular and earned a commanding position in the fragrance world.

COLOGNE a toilet water originating in the 18th century in the city of Cologne; now also a lighter version of a scent or perfume.

ENFLEURAGE the French method of extracting scent from flowers by forcing the flowers to yield their scent to purified cold fat; this is washed in alcohol and the alcohol distilled to extract the scent.

ESSENTIAL OILS the oils extracted by distillation.

FIXATIVE a substance that holds the more volatile ingredients, keeping them stable and harmonious. Can be either synthetic or the natural animal fixatives such as musk, civet, ambergris and castoreum.

FLORAL OR FLOWERY a scent smelling of flowers. Single florals evoke the scent of a single flower, although they may have a complicated blend of ingredients. Floral *bouquets*, or flowery scents, are a blend of several flowers, often combined with other ingredients, where the flowery notes are strongest. Often very sweet.

FRUITY a blend in which the sweet heavy smells of fruits like peach, quince, pineapple and passion-fruit are dominant.

GRASSE the ancient hill town in the South of France, renowned as the centre of the French perfume industry. This is where the *essential oils* and *absolutes* are coaxed from flowers, herbs, roots, spices, leaves and woods – some grown locally, many imported – then blended into famous and new perfumes.

GREEN a fresh, clean scent usually containing ingredients like pine, fern, moss, grass, flower stems and leaves, plus citrus.

HERBAL a scent in which the smell of rosemary, mint or lavender, for instance, is especially strong.

HYACINTH Madame de Pompadour's favourite perfume; so expensive that only the very rich could afford it. Now it is included in many *floral* or 'spring flower' blends.

INCENSE burning oil. A very ancient method of perfuming the atmosphere – modern versions include joss sticks, rings filled with oil to place on the light bulb and candles.

JASMINE a most valuable ingredient, second only to the rose, found in the majority of great scents and obtained from the white, intensely scented flower.

KYPHI the fabulous ancient Egyptian perfume, made famous by Cleopatra, probably made from herbs and resins like myrrh, spikenard and henna with fruits such as raisins.

LINGER the lasting quality or staying power provided by *fixatives* and possessed by most recently created scents.

MODERN a blend using primarily synthetic ingredients – floral, *green*, herbal, warm, *spicy* or unidentifiable.

MUSK a *fixative* derived from a glandular secretion of the musk deer found in Tibet and much prized for its erotic, lasting powers. It is said to have been worn by the Empress Joséphine and to have lingered in her rooms long after her death.

NOSE a master *parfumeur* whose sense of smell is so highly

developed and pure that he can not only recognize and 'break down' ingredients in existing scents but still create truly original new blends.

ORANGE FLOWER an ingredient from the sweet orange tree – a popular flower, found in many old and new scents, with an intoxicating smell, symbolic of youth and brides. Neroli, from the bitter orange tree, has a dryer fresher scent.

ORIENTAL a rich, warm variety of scent usually containing balsams, resins from aromatic Eastern woods and plants, musk, ambergris and the heavier flower scents – tuberose, gardenia, jasmine.

OTTO OR ATTAR a concentrated distilled essence, usually of the rose.

PATCHOULI an oil derived from the leaves of an East Indian plant with a dry, haunting odour not unlike pencil shavings. Often associated with cashmere shawls in the Victorian era.

ROOTS ingredients such as iris (or orris) root, which provides the scent of violets in many perfumes; also vetiver grass.

ROSE the flower most of whose many varieties – musk rose, tea rose, etc. – produce a sweet smell; most prized of all is the Bulgarian rose, without which few perfumes would exist today as they are. Precious and expensive – half a ton of petals must be crushed to make one pound of rose attar. The scent of roses was loved by Elizabeth I, whose ladies in waiting made rosewater wherever her court was assembled.

SANDALWOOD a scent from the wood of a parasitic tree that attaches itself to the roots of other trees – found mostly in India and Australia.

SPICE a variety of perfume heavier than *floral* but not as heavy as the *Oriental* types. Usually a blend of exotic flowers with spices like clove, ginger and cinnamon.

SYNTHETICS the fragrant inventions that emerge from laboratories – enormously useful in creating new perfumes and preventing prices from soaring even higher.

TOP NOTE the smell you smell first, before the perfume has warmed on your skin and revealed the middle notes or remained on long enough to produce the base.

TUBEROSE a flower (no relation to the rose) which produces an intoxicating, distinctive fragrance.

VARIETIES the categories, also known as divisions or kinds, into which most scents are divided, e.g. *floral, green, Oriental, fruity, chypre.*

VETIVER a superb *essential oil* from the roots of an aromatic grass found in the islands of the Indian Ocean.

VIOLET both the flowers and leaves are valuable to perfumery but very difficult to extract. However, iris (or orris) root provides a similar smell. Violets were the favourite flower of the Empress Joséphine.

X that added quality that comes from your own chemistry and skin and warms to your personality.

YLANG YLANG the scent with a poignant bitter-sweet quality from the flower of the same name. It means 'flower of flowers' to the South Sea Islanders.

ZANZIBAR the place where spice markets abound and the air is redolent with the scent of cloves.

Do's and Don'ts

DON'T mix scent with the sun. Some ingredients, when exposed to skin and sun, can cause allergies, rashes or brown patches. So, if you are spending time outside in hot sun, on the beach or water or skiing in the mountains, keep your fragrance for evening allure. Do store scent in a dark, cool place. Light can cause chemical reaction and change the nature of the fragrance. If it's well sealed and well stored, it will last about a year and still be true – unsealed, exposed to light and heat, it oxidizes and deteriorates quite fast. DON'T try more than three scents at the same time when you're contemplating something new. This is about as many as the average nose can accept before becoming tired. Spray or dab a little on the inside of the wrist, do the same on the other wrist and try the back of one hand for the third. Wait a minute or so for each one to develop, then smell it before applying the next. And, don't make your final decision before smelling them all again half an hour later.

Do think of fragrance in a much wider context than just its original bottle. Investigate the possibilities of having eau de toilette (splash it on during the day and keep the more concentrated version for evening), bath oil, body lotion, talcum powder, soap, deodorant. And, look out for other accessories in the same fragrance – candles, coat-hangers, drawer sachets, room sprays, so that everything about you smells the same.

DON'T try and transfer your favourite scent to a plastic bottle for travelling – it tends to evaporate through plastic and you may lose it all. Travel with a purse spray or a small sealed bottle that's not plastic.

Do try spraying your ironing board with fragrance before ironing shirts and dresses.

DON'T waste your scent on the air instead of on you. Once a bottle has been opened, use it – it will only evaporate and lose its potency if you try to save it.

Tessa Traeger

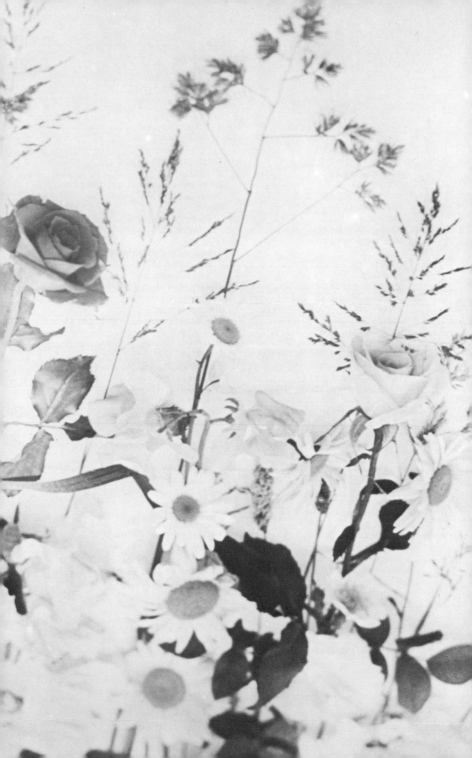

Index